Infection Control
A Handbook for Community Nurses

Infection Control

A Handbook for Community Nurses

HARSH V. DUGGAL MBBS, LMSSA, FFPHM
Consultant in Communicable Disease Control,
South Staffordshire Health Authority

AMANDA M. BEAUMONT RGN, MPH
Clinical Nurse Specialist – Infection Control,
South Staffordshire Health Authority

and
HELEN J. JENKINSON RGN, DPSN
Clinical Nurse Specialist – Infection Control,
South Staffordshire Health Authority

SERIES EDITOR
MARILYN EDWARDS BSc(Hons), SRN, FETC
Specialist Practitioner, General Practice Nursing,
Bilbrook Medical Centre, Staffordshire

W
WHURR PUBLISHERS
LONDON AND PHILADELPHIA

© 2002 Whurr Publishers
Pennsylvania

First published 2002 by
Whurr Publishers Ltd
19b Compton Terrace, London N1 2UN, England
325 Chestnut Street, Philadelphia PA 19106, USA

British Library Cataloguing in Publication Data

A catalogue record for this book is available from the British
Library.

ISBN 1 86156 255 1

Printed and bound in the UK by Athenaeum Press Limited,
Gateshead, Tyne & Wear.

Contents

Foreword

Infection poses a major challenge to health-care staff. It is a common cause of morbidity, and not infrequent cause of mortality, both in hospital and in the community. The medico-legal implications of infection are an increasing challenge and advisory documents and regulations relating to control of infectious diseases arrive regularly from various offical organizations such as the Health and Safety Executive and the National Health Service.

The authors of this book are to be congratulated on writing a handbook on infection control for community nurses who are frequently in the frontline of infectious disease management. The question and answer format of the text is clear and practical and addresses most of the frequently asked questions about common infections.

I commend the handbook to community nurses and, indeed, to nurses in general.

Professor Alasdair Geddes
CBE, FRCP, FRCPath, FFPHM, FMedSci
School of Medicine, University of Birmingham

Series Preface

This series of handbooks has been devised to help community nurses answer commonly asked questions. Many of the questions are asked by patients, others by colleagues. The books have been written by specialists, and although they are not intended as full clinical texts, they are fully referenced from current evidence to validate the content. The purpose of each handbook is to provide 'facts at the fingertips', so that trawling through textbooks is not needed. This is achieved through the question and answer format, with cross-referencing between sections. Where further information may be required, the reader is referred to specific texts. Many patients want some control over their illnesses, and use the internet to access information. The useful address sections include website addresses to share with both patients and colleagues.

It is hoped that these handy reference books will answer most every-day questions. If there are areas which you feel have been neglected, please let us know for future editions.

Mandy Edwards

Introduction

Communicable diseases have been around for hundreds of years. As success is achieved in reducing infections – measles, haemophilus influenzae type B meningitis – new diseases have emerged, such as cryptosporidiosis, *E. coli* 0157, human immunodeficiency virus, hepatitis C, new variant Creutzfeldt-Jakob disease, and have become important public health problems. Communicable diseases feature regularly in the media, especially food-related illnesses. One of the main ways of educating the public is to make them aware of communicable diseases, such as salmonella in eggs, listeria in soft cheeses and bovine spongiform encephalopathy in cattle. Although infections usually cause morbidity, deaths do occur but are rare, with the exceptions of meningitis in children and complications of influenza in the elderly. In developing countries, however, infections are an important cause of premature death.

Ill health caused by infections should be the concern of all those with responsibilities for the control of communicable diseases. Effective public health strategies against communicable diseases depend upon surveillance, preventive measures, outbreak investigation, and institution of control of measures including appropriate treatment. This book describes some common and other important communicable diseases likely to be encountered by community nurses. It offers community nurses practical solutions to manage patients presenting with infections.

Infection control in the community starts with staff hygiene and a clean environment, which are described in Chapter 1. Chapter 2 examines causes and management of blood-borne illnesses, which are a major concern within certain client groups.

Although not usually fatal, gastrointestinal infections can result in severe morbidity. Chapter 3 examines the common infections and their management within the public health arena. Community nurses are frequently asked for advice about parasitic infections, which although not life threatening cause distress to sufferers and their parents/carers. Recommendations for current treatment of head lice, scabies and thread-worms are explained in Chapter 4.

Cases of respiratory tuberculosis (TB) are increasing in the United Kingdom, although they are more commonly found in certain client groups. Influenza (and especially prevention of influenza) creates a massive workload for community staff every autumn and winter. The role of the community nurse in prevention and care of people suffering from TB and influenza is discussed in Chapter 5.

Other common infections are discussed in Chapter 6. The reader is referred to Appendix 1 for information on incubation periods for child-hood illnesses.

This handbook has been written in a question-and-answer format for ease of reference, with topics cross-referenced where appropriate. This will enable readers to have the answers to common questions at their fingertips.

Chapter 1
The environment

Introduction

Prevention and control of infection is fundamental to the provision of a safe environment for patients and forms an integral part of the practice of any healthcare professional working in a clinical setting (Wilson, 1995). This chapter will explain the safe practices recommended to reduce infection in the community. The treatment room includes anywhere that treatment is undertaken in a clinical area. The home includes private homes and residential establishments.

The treatment room

Q1.1 What are the important issues relating to the treatment room?

Within general practice it is important that the clinical area should be well organized and separated into clean and dirty zones to prevent cross-contamination.

Work surfaces in clinical rooms and couches should be made of materials that are easily cleaned with detergent (washing-up liquid) and water.

Surfaces such as walls, floors and furniture do not come into contact with the patient and are a low infection risk. Therefore basic decontamination/cleaning with detergent and water is sufficient.

Examination couches should be covered with a disposable paper sheet, which should be changed after each patient use. This is sufficient for hygiene purposes, and the couch can be easily wiped with detergent and water if contamination occurs, and at the end of each surgery session. Cover blankets to maintain a patient's dignity, if required, should be small and easily washable and changed between patients.

The treatment room should be used for clinical procedures and for storage of sterile and clean equipment only. Used or contaminated products should not be stored there. All sterile products should be stored above floor level and preferably in cupboards to keep them dust free and to prevent them being splashed, and/or packaging being torn. An area should be provided for the safe disposal of body fluids and storage of dirty equipment. Specimens must not be disposed of down a sink but should be thrown away in accordance with the Duty of Care (Environmental Protection Act 1990 – published 1996) either down a sluice, lavatory or in a container and into clinical waste bags (see Q1.11).

Q1.2 Why is the importance of hand washing always stressed?

To reduce the transmission of infection it is vital that the hands of all healthcare workers are clean, washed regularly and that the hand-washing technique is of a high standard (Wilson, 1995). Hand washing remains the single most important infection control measure. One method of hand washing is described in Figure 1.1 (Ayliffe et al., 1992).

In the primary healthcare setting there are many procedures undertaken in one area, usually the treatment room, as it is very rare for practice premises to have separate clinical rooms for minor surgery, well-men clinics or wound dressing. It is therefore important that hand-washing facilities are conveniently located within the clinical area.

The resources within a general practice setting used for hand washing must not create a risk of cross-infection, therefore hand-washing facilities must be separate from the sink used to wash instruments and must be well maintained. Poorly cleaned and maintained hand basins and soap dispensers may create a cross-infection risk (Bowell, 1992). Ideally, elbow taps should be available at the hand-washing sink.

It is equally important to wash hands after contact with a patient in his/her own home. To wash hands in a home environment:

1. Use the patient's water and soap facilities if available.
2. Keep a supply of disposable paper hand towels with you to dry your hands. Do not use the patient's hand towel as this may be heavily contaminated. Dispose of the paper towel in the patient's own refuse.
3. If a patient's facilities are such that you are unable to wash your hands using the patient's facilities, then a hand sanitizer containing alcohol should be used.

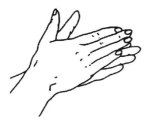
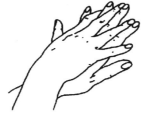
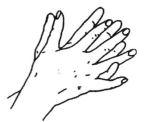

1. Palm to palm

2. Right palm over left dorsum, left palm over right dorsum

3. Palm to palm, fingers interlaced

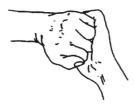
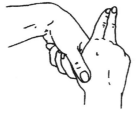
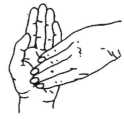

4. Back of fingers to opposing with fingers interlaced

5. Rotational rubbing of right thumb clasped over left palm

6. Rotational rubbing backwards and forewards with fingers of right hand in palm of left, and vice versa

1. Sufficient soap (liquid) should be applied to the hands to obtain a good lather. Hands should always be washed under warm running water. Hand-washing techniques, regardless of the product selected, must ensure that no area of skin surface is missed during the procedure.
2. Rub the hands as shown in Figure 1.1.
3. Rinse.
4. Dry thoroughly using disposable paper towels.

Source: Ayliffe et al. (1992).

Figure 1.1 Hand washing.

Q1.3 When should hands be washed?

- after handling blood and body fluids;
- before aseptic techniques;
- before handling or eating food;
- after each patient contact.

Q1.4 When should gloves be worn?

Since the development of universal precautions in 1988 (DOH 1998a), designed to protect healthcare workers from risks arising from contact with blood and body fluids, the glove has become an essential piece of equipment to the healthcare worker. Gloves should be worn to:

- protect the user from handling infectious material, i.e. blood, faeces, urine;
- protect the client from transient micro-organisms;
- minimize cross-infections, thereby protecting nurse and client.

Gloves are recommended to be worn when in direct contact with blood or body fluids and for direct contact with non-intact skin or mucous membranes. Sterile surgical gloves should be used for procedures involving contact with normally sterile areas of the body.

Non-sterile vinyl gloves should be used for procedures involving contact with mucous membranes or any procedures where contact with body excretions or secretions is likely.

Always change gloves between patients and wash hands even though gloves have been worn.

Do not wash or disinfect gloves for reuse. This can cause penetration of liquids through undetected holes and may cause deterioration.

Plastic gloves are not recommended for use in a healthcare setting as they are porous and offer no protection from body fluids. These are supplied with a paper backing, and are uncommonly found in doctors' surgeries. They have no place as a current infection control measure.

Q1.5 How should body fluid spillage be removed?

Always wear a plastic apron and disposable gloves before handling any body fluids. Box 1.1 lists the management of body spillage.

Box 1.1 Management of body spillage	
Spillage	*Management*
Urine	Clean with general-purpose detergent and dry area thoroughly
Faeces/vomit	Wipe up spillage with disposable paper towel. Clean the area using soap and water and dry thoroughly
Blood	Ensure good ventilation
	Use chlorine granules to soak up the blood and wipe up with a paper towel
	Wash area with bleach-based product diluted to 1000 ppm available chlorine
	Dry area thoroughly If area carpeted, do not use bleach product; instead soak up spill with paper towels, clean with detergent carpet shampoo and steam clean area as soon as possible Carpets are not recommended in the clinical room

Q1.6 How are sharps disposed of in the practice?

Safe disposal of sharp instruments is the responsibility of the user. Sharp instruments can cause injury to healthcare workers and therefore should be handled with care and disposed of safely (BSI, 1990). Box 1.2 lists general rules for sharps disposal.

Box 1.2 General rules for sharps disposal

Needles should not be resheathed

Discard syringe and needle as one unit into a recommended sharps container

Never leave sharps to be disposed of by someone else

Sharps containers should be sealed and labelled with the name of the practice and discarded when they are no more than three-quarters full (and must never be placed in a yellow clinical waste bag)

All sharps must be disposed of by incineration

Sharps containers must comply with BS 7320 and UN3291 (BSI, 1990)

Sharps boxes in use should be positioned out of reach of patients

Take bin to sharp, not sharp to bin

Minor Surgery in General Practice

Minor surgical operations have been part of general practice for many years. Prior to 1990 and the GP minor surgery scheme only 25 per cent of GPs carried out minor surgical procedures in their practices (HSG (93) 40 – revised 1996).

Q1.7 How should the room be prepared for minor surgery?

Clean and dirty areas should be clearly defined to reduce the risk of cross-infection and all surfaces should be impermeable and easy to clean (see Q1.1). More thorough hand washing is necessary than for general procedures – see Box 1.3 (page 6).

Q1.8 What equipment is needed to reduce the risk of infection during minor surgery?

Recommended equipment is detailed in Box 1.4.

Q1.9 What preparation does the patient require?

The aim of disinfecting skin sites prior to surgery is to remove and reduce the number of resident bacteria. The preparation used should be fast

---

Box 1.3 Minor surgery infection control – hand washing

The sink should be fitted with a mixer tap, elbow operated

There should be a supply of liquid soap and disposable paper towels next to the sink

If nailbrushes are used they should be single use; repeated scrubbing with nailbrushes will damage the skin and may be associated with an increase in resident bacteria on the surface of the skin

Before the first surgical case hands and forearms should be washed thoroughly with soap and water for two minutes

NB: Antiseptic detergent hand-wash preparations are usually chlorhexidine or iodine based Surgical hand disinfection should be carried out prior to performing any minor surgery

A separate deep sink is recommended for the washing of instruments

---

Box 1.4 Equipment for the clinical room/undertaking minor surgery

Hand cleansers (see Q1.4)

Paper towels (see Q1.4)

Sharps bin (see Q1.6)

Sterile gloves (see Q1.10)

Aprons (see Q1.10)

Yellow clinical waste bag (see Q1.11)

Foot-controlled waste bin (see Q1.11)

Trolley (sterile area)

Bench-top autoclave – to sterilize equipment at point of use (see Q1.13)

Or sterile packs (available from hospital sterile supply department)

Or disposable sterile instruments/sterile metal instruments (see Q1.12)

---

acting and have a prolonged antibacterial effect. The skin-cleansing solution (e.g. iodine, chlorhexidine and alcohol) should be applied liberally to the site and surrounding area, then allowed to dry. Skin disinfection should be carried out immediately prior to surgery.

Q 1.10 What personal protective equipment (PPE) is required in minor surgery?

The practice nurse assisting in minor surgical procedures should wear a disposable plastic apron; sterile surgical gloves should be used for any procedure involving contact with normally sterile areas of the body. Both should be disposed of as clinical waste (DoH, 1998a; Health and Safety Executive, 1992). Goggles should be worn if there is a potential risk of splashing.

Q1.11 What is the correct clinical waste procedure?

Clinical waste should always be placed in a foot-operated waste bin with a lid (see Table 6.1, Q6.11). Yellow clinical waste bags should be removed at the end of each session/day and placed in the designated holding area for clinical waste in accordance with the Duty of Care (HSAC, 1999).

It is essential that domestic staff who deal with clinical waste are aware of health and safety procedures for dealing with clinical waste.

Q1.12 What methods of cleaning, disinfection and sterilization are recommended in general practice?

General practitioners are responsible for the effective operation and maintenance of sterilizing equipment in their practices (HSG (93) 40 – revised 1996). However, it is often the practice nurse who is most familiar with the day-to-day workings of the equipment and the day-to-day function tests (see Q1.13).

Cleaning the treatment room and the equipment used

It is important that staff understand what they are trying to achieve when they clean, disinfect or sterilize instruments or equipment. Table 1.1 defines the different activities.

Table 1.1 Definition of activities

Cleaning
Removal of organic matter: essential process prior to disinfection or sterilization
It can be achieved, usually, using hot water and washing-up liquid
The use of chlorhexidine-based hand washes to clean instruments is not recommended — it is expensive and unnecessary

Disinfection
Reduction of viable micro-organisms — but this may not inactivate bacterial spores and some viruses.

Sterilization
Destruction of all viable micro-organisms including bacterial spores

Q1.13 What are the methods of sterilization?

Some practices choose to own a sterilizer within the practice and therefore must be responsible for its management and maintenance. There are alternatives to each practice owning a sterilizer. Some practices may decide that they wish to use disposable sterile equipment; others may be able to make arrangements to send their instruments for sterilization to the local hospital sterile supplies department, which will provide a service for them.

If it is decided that the practice does wish to purchase a sterilizer then the equipment should be correctly maintained and monitored to ensure effective sterilization. The Health Technical Memorandum 2010 (DoH, 1994) is regarded as the authoritative work on sterilization and applies to all bench-top sterilizers. The aim of the guidance is to ensure the efficiency and safety of a sterilizer. Proper procedures and maintenance of the machine help to ensure that instruments are sterilized. The memorandum outlines the responsibilities of those involved in purchasing, buying and maintaining a sterilizer. The user is responsible for the management of the sterilizer, and whether it is fit for use.

Tests should be carried out each day, or if the sterilizer is used infrequently, the tests should be done prior to use (see Box 1.5).

Box 1.5 Daily sterilizer check

1. Wipe out/clean sterilizer chamber
2. Check/clean door seal, in accordance with local procedures/manufacturer's instructions
3. Check/fill water reservoir
4. Run cycle and note:

   - temperature 134°C minimum when sterilizing
   - pressure 2.2 bar minimum when sterilizing
   - sterilization hold time 3.0–3.5 minutes
   - total cycle time 15 minutes

5. Visual check for leaks or anything unusual
6. Record number of cycles where possible
7. Complete and sign the user record sheet

In the event of a breakdown, inform the maintenance engineer

Sterilizer user test record

Test	1	2	3	4a	4b	4c	4d	5	6	7
Date	Clean chamber	Check door	Check water	Check 134°C	Check 2.2 bar	Check 3.0–3.5 min hold	Check & time 15 min	Check leaks	Record cycles	Print name
1.1.01	✓	✓	✓	✓	✓	✓	✓	✓	2	A.Non
2.1.01	✓	✓	✓	✓	✓	✓	✓	✓	1	A.Non

Source: Adapted from HTM 2010 (DoH, 1994).

The practice also needs to ensure that more thorough maintenance is carried out in accordance with HTM 2010 (DoH, 1994). A company qualified to do such work can carry out the necessary tests, and there should always be a record of all the tests and maintenance carried out on the machine so that the practice can demonstrate that the regulations have been complied with. Some sterilizers can produce a printed record of the sterilization process, which should be considered if traceability of records is required; this can then be attached to the patient's notes if he/she has undergone minor surgery within the practice.

The use of chemical disinfectants is governed by Control of Substances Hazardous to Health regulations (HSE, 1994), which have strict guidelines on the use of chemicals such as glutaraldehyde. The use of glutaraldehyde can expose staff to serious health risks. Adequate facilities such as fume cupboards and personal protective equipment must be available. Staff using glutaraldehyde, even under controlled conditions, should have their health monitored by an occupational health department or equivalent (HSE, 1994).

Q1.14 What are universal precautions?

As it is not always possible to identify people who are infectious to others as opposed to those who are not, basic infection control principles and procedures must be adopted for each and every individual.

The aim of these 'universal precautions' is to protect both carer and client from the transmission of infection during hazardous procedures when the risk is known or unknown (see Box 1.6, page 10). These precautions ensure maximum protection without the need to divulge information that may be confidential.

Q1.15 Are there any special guidelines for the storage of vaccines?

It is essential that vaccines are stored according to the recommended storage guidelines, to maintain their potency and effectiveness (Box 1.7, page 10).

Q1.16 How should communally used devices be cleaned?

Awareness of the need for good infection control practice is essential. Never before has infection control been so high profile than since the emergence of the Department of Health guidance on the decontamination of medical devices (HSC, 1999/178; HSC, 1999/179; HSC, 2000/032) (Box 1.8).

Box 1.6 Universal precautions

Apply good basic hygiene practices with regular hand washing (see Q1.2)

Avoid contamination by appropriate use of protective clothing (see Q1.4, Q1.5)

Protect mucous membrane, eyes, mouth and nose from blood spillages (see Q1.5)

Avoid sharps usage wherever possible (see Box 1.2)

Cover all cuts and grazes with waterproof dressings (plaster)

Wear disposable non-sterile vinyl gloves if handling blood or body fluids (see Q1.5)

Disposable items soiled with blood or body fluids should be disposed of in yellow clinical waste bags, not black bin bags (see Q1.11)

All blood, faeces and vomit spills must be cleaned up promptly using a blood spillage kit (see Box 1.1)

Urine spills can be cleaned up using general purpose detergent — DO NOT USE A BLOOD SPILLAGE KIT (see Box 1.1)

Institute approved procedures for sterilization and disinfection of instruments and equipment (see Q1.12, Q1.16)

Box 1.7 Vaccine storage

All vaccine fridges should have a maximum and minimum thermometer in order to keep a regular check on the temperature of the fridge. Most vaccines should be stored between 2° and 8° Celsius

A temperature check should be done daily and recorded by a designated person. A temperature check should also be undertaken prior to vaccination clinics and recorded by a designated person. If on recording the temperature the maximum or minimum temperature is too high or too low it should be reported immediately and the manufacturer or local pharmacist contacted for further advice on usage

The thermometer should be reset after the temperature check has been performed

The vaccine fridge should be defrosted regularly and when defrosting alternative arrangements should be made for storage of vaccines. This could be a cool box with appropriate cooling blocks

The vaccine fridge should be used for storing vaccines only. No food or specimens should be stored with vaccines

Vaccines should not touch the sides of the fridge or be packed too tightly together

Vaccines should always be transported in a cool box for home visits

Vaccines should not be allowed to freeze

Box 1.8 Decontamination of devices		
High risk	Devices that come into direct contact with mucous membranes, broken skin or sterile body cavities/areas, e.g. surgical instruments	These items must be sterile at the point of use
Medium risk	Devices that come into contact with mucous membranes with easily transmissible or virulent organisms, e.g. speculae	These items need not be sterile at the point of use, but must be sterilized after use
Low risk	Devices that come into contact with intact skin or mucous membranes, e.g. auroscope ends	These items require thorough cleaning with detergent and water

The Medical Devices Agency 2000 clearly identifies that items marked for single patient use/single use must not be reused in any circumstances, for example nebulisers (HSC 2000).

Q1.17 How should specimens be stored and which ones can be stored overnight?

As a general principle, specimens should be sent to the laboratory as soon as possible. Stool specimens can be stored overnight as long as they are kept in the fridge. Urine and sputum specimens should ideally reach the laboratory within four hours. However, they can be kept overnight in the fridge, although any specimens over 24 hours old are not acceptable. Specimens should not be stored in a vaccine fridge.

Summary

General principles in infection control are based on the use of practices and procedures that prevent or reduce the likelihood of infections being transmitted from a source of infection (e.g. person, contaminated body fluid, equipment, etc.) to a susceptible host (Department of Health 1998a).

Chapter 2
Blood-borne infections

Introduction

Blood-borne infections are a major public health concern, causing severe morbidity and premature mortality for sufferers.

Hepatitis is a generic term indicating inflammation of the liver. Viruses are the commonest cause of hepatitis but there are other causes, such as drugs and alcohol.

Acute viral hepatitis is a systemic infection affecting mainly the liver. Six different viral agents have been isolated: Hepatitis A virus (HAV), Hepatitis B virus (HBV), Hepatitis C virus (HCV), Hepatitis D virus (HDV), Hepatitis E virus (HEV) and Hepatitis G virus (HGV). Although the mode of transmission may be blood borne (HBV, HCV, HDV, HGV) or food borne (HAV, HEV) they all produce clinically similar illness, which may vary from asymptomatic or subclinical disease to fulminating and fatal acute infections. For HAV see Q3.6 to Q3.27.

The human immunodeficiency virus (HIV) was first identified in 1981 and has caused the deaths of millions of people around the world. There is no vaccine available to prevent HIV infection and although there have been some developments in therapy as yet there is no cure for AIDS. The aetiology and management of the more common blood-borne diseases will be examined in this chapter, with emphasis on infection control in the community.

Hepatitis B

Q2.1 What is Hepatitis B (HBV)?

Hepatitis B is an infectious disease caused by a blood-borne virus that was identified in the 1960s.

Q2.2 How common is HBV?

HBV is a global disease. The highest incidence of the disease is in Southeast Asia and Africa, the lowest in Europe and North America. In England and Wales there are between 500 and 600 new cases reported annually (Mangtani et al., 1998). The number of new infections has remained the same in the 1990s but has shown an upward trend in the past few years.

Q2.3 What is the incubation period?

The incubation period can range from four weeks to six months with an average of around three months.

Q2.4 How is HBV transmitted?

HBV is present in virtually all body fluids, although only blood, saliva, vaginal fluid, breast milk and semen have been found to be infective (Teo, 1992). The three main ways of transmission are:

1. inoculation of blood or body fluids from one person to another;
2. sexual intercourse;
3. transmission of infection from mother to baby at birth.

Q2.5 Who is most at risk of getting HBV infection?

Anybody can get HBV infection although there are some specific patterns. In those countries where the incidence is high the most common route of transmission is from mother to baby. In developed countries within Europe exposure to infection mainly takes place in adults, of which those at most risk are intravenous drug abusers, homosexual men, heterosexuals with multiple partners and healthcare staff (Mangtani et al., 1998).

Q2.6 What are the symptoms of HBV?

The severity of disease varies widely and many infections are inapparent (Chin, 2000). Asymptomatic patients may be identified through abnormal liver function tests (see Q2.11). Box 2.1 lists symptoms for those with a clinical illness.

Box 2.1 Symptoms of Hepatitis B

Onset is usually insidious with headache, malaise, loss of appetite, nausea and vomiting

Fever appears about a week before the onset of jaundice in icteric cases

Often there is aversion to food and tobacco

Urine becomes dark and stools light or clay coloured

Clinical illness may be undistinguishable from Hepatitis A. In a small number of patients there may be fatal fulminatory liver infection

---

Q2.7 What is the natural history of HBV?

Of those who are exposed to infection as adults 90–95 per cent will recover fully and a small number (5–10 per cent) will become chronic carriers of the disease. In time, some of them will go on to develop chronic hepatitis, cirrhosis or liver cancer. When infection is acquired at birth the disease is often asymptomatic but nearly 90 per cent develop long-term carrier status (DOH, 1996a). Chronic carrier status varies from 1 to 2 per 1000 in the UK to nearly 10 per cent in some Asian/African countries.

Q2.8 How long is a person infectious to others?

HBV is infectious during the latter part of the incubation period and through the acute clinical course of the disease – usually a period of about six months. A small number of those who get infection (5–10 per cent) end up as chronic carriers (see Q2.7). They are potentially infectious throughout life although they may have no symptoms themselves.

Q2.9 Can you get HBV many times?

No, once you have had the infection you will have immunity against the disease for the rest of your life.

Q2.10 How is HBV diagnosed?

As for any other disease, there are three elements:

1. a history of exposure (this is not always easily obtainable);
2. clinical symptoms and signs – see Box 2.1;
3. laboratory investigations – see Q2.11.

Q2.11 Are there any specific laboratory tests for HBV?

Most people will present following an illness that leads to jaundice, and laboratory tests for liver functions would be abnormal, indicating hepatitis. The diagnostic test for HBV is based on the detection of three serological markers in the blood of patients. The virus is composed of a nucleocapsid core, surrounded by an outer protein containing the surface antigen. The third marker of HBV infection 'e' antigen is found in soluble forms in virus-positive sera and is related to the core antigen (Box 2.2).

Box 2.2 Hepatitis B markers	
Antigens	*Antibodies*
Surface antigen (HBs Ag)	Antibody to surface antigen (Anti HBs)
Found in the latter part of incubation period and acute phase of HBV infection. Patients remaining HBs Ag positive for more then six months are regarded as having developed the chronic carrier state and are potentially infectious	In those recovering from natural infection this is associated with the disappearance of infectious virus. Antibodies also develop in response to HBV immunization. When present in adequate titre confers immunity
Core antigen (HBcAg)	Core antibody (Anti HBc)
This does not circulate in serum and is confined to infected cells	This indicates exposure to HBV infections either recent (Igm) or previous (Igg)
HBe antigen (HBeAg)	Antibody to HBe (Anti HBe)
When present indicates active viral replication and HBeAg positive blood is highly infectious	Presence usually denotes cessation of active viral replication and anti-HBe carrier's blood is potentially less infectious

Q2.12 How is HBV treated?

Most people who suffer an acute attack will need supportive nursing and medical care. Specific treatment for HBV may be necessary for people in whom the virus persists for more than six months, i.e. chronic carrier status (see Q2.8). These patients can be referred to specialist liver units for regular monitoring to determine whether treatment is necessary. Those who need treatment receive the drug interferon alpha. In approximately half of the people treated with interferon, hepatitis will be converted from highly infectious to mildly infectious and inflammation of the liver will improve. Patients who are exposed to the virus at birth tend to respond less well to interferon treatment (see Q2.7).

Q2.13 How can HBV be prevented?

HBV can be prevented by reducing blood and body fluid contact between an infected and a non-infected person. Blood for transfusion in the United Kingdom is screened for HBV and has been safe for many years. Organ donors are also screened for HBV. Screening of antenatal women will identify those who are chronic carriers so that action can be taken to prevent infection in the baby (DoH, 1998b) by providing hepatitis B immunoglobulin with vaccine at birth (see Q2.14). Appropriate infection control procedures in healthcare settings have helped to reduce transmission between patients and healthcare staff and vice versa (see Q1.11, Q1.13, Box 1.2).

Other measures, such as practising safer sex and not sharing needles and syringes, would go a long way to preventing the disease. Experience to date is that HBV is much more infectious than the Hepatitis C virus or human immunodeficiency virus.

There is a vaccine that can be given to prevent HBV (see Q2.14).

Q2.14 How does HBV vaccine prevent infection?

There are two ways of preventing HBV by the use of vaccine (DoH, 1996a).

Passive immunity by an injection of Hepatitis B immunoglobulin (HBIG – the antibodies) can be given to those at risk. HBIG is in short supply and is indicated only in the following situations (PHLS, 1992).

- babies born to mothers who have acute hepatitis B during pregnancy or who are chronic carriers;
- persons who are accidentally inoculated or contaminated in the eye, mouth, fresh cuts or abrasions of the skin, with the blood from an HBs Ag positive person (see Box 2.2).
- sexual partners of individuals suffering from acute hepatitis B, who are seen within one week of onset of jaundice in the infected person.

Supplies of HBIG are available from the local Public Health Laboratories Service. A single dose of HBIG (normally 500 iu for adults; 200 iu for the newborn) is sufficient and should preferably be given within 48 hours of exposure.

The second way of preventing HBV infection is by injecting a vaccine that produces an immune response. The vaccine is effective in preventing infection in individuals who produce specific antibodies to the hepatitis B surface antigen. Overall 80–90 per cent of individuals have a response to the vaccine. Those over the age of 40 are less likely to respond. Patients who are immunodeficient or on immunosuppressive therapy respond less well than healthy individuals and may require larger doses of vaccine or an additional dose.

The basic immunization regimen consists of three doses of vaccine:

- the first dose is given on the elected day;
- the second dose one month later;
- the third dose six months after the first dose.

Sometimes it is necessary to have an accelerated schedule for more rapid immunization, when the third dose may be given at two months after the initial dose with a booster dose at 12 months (DoH, 1996a). The vaccine should normally be given intramuscularly in the deltoid region, although the anterolateral thigh is the preferred site in infants. There are at present two licensed products and the manufacturer's dosage schedule should be adhered to.

Two months following completion of the course, the surface antibody level should be checked for response. A level of 10 iu/ml or more is considered protective and those below 10 iu/ml are not immune. The duration of antibody response is not precisely known at present. A booster five years after completing the primary course is recommended to retain immunity. Once adequate antibody response is documented following the primary course there is no need to test blood again before giving a booster at five years.

The vaccine should not be given to individuals who have acute Hepatitis B disease or those who are known to be surface antigen positive, as in the former case it is unnecessary and in the latter it is ineffective (see Box 2.2).

Q2.15 Who should be given Hepatitis B vaccine?

The World Health Organisation policy aimed to introduce universal immunization within the childhood programme throughout the world by 1997 (Van Damme, 1997). In the UK the policy at present is to immunize only those at risk, who include (Department of Health 1996a):

1. babies born to mothers who have had acute HBV infection in pregnancy or are chronic carriers of HBV (See Q2.5–2.8);

2. parenteral drug misusers (See Q2.5);
3. individuals who change sexual partners frequently (See Q2.5);
4. close family contacts of a case or carrier;
5. families adopting children from countries with high prevalence of Hepatitis B (see Q2.2);
6. haemophiliacs;
7. patients with chronic renal failure;
8. healthcare workers who have direct contact with patients' blood or bloodstained body fluids (see Q2.13, 2.16);
9. staff and residents of residential accommodation for those with severe learning disabilities;
10. other staff who are at risk because of their occupation;
11. inmates of custodial institutions;
12. those travelling to areas of high prevalence (see Q2.2, Q2.17).

Q2.16 Should all healthcare workers be immunized against Hepatitis B?

It would depend on the risk of exposure (DoH, 1993). Staff who are going to be involved with procedures involving blood and body fluids should protect themselves (see Q1.10, Box 1.2). There are well-documented outbreaks associated with infected surgeons (Heptonstall, 1992). It is clear, therefore, that surgeons should be immunized. For others it is a matter of making an assessment of risk.

Q2.17 What are the implications for travellers?

Short-term tourists or business travellers are not generally in increased danger of infection unless they place themselves at risk by their sexual behaviour when abroad. They need to be advised on safe sex while abroad.

Those travelling to areas of high prevalence who intend to seek employment as healthcare workers or those who plan to remain there for lengthy periods and who may therefore be at increased risk of acquiring infection as a result of medical and dental procedures carried out in those countries should be protected with Hepatitis B vaccine (see Q2.14).

Q2.18 If a patient is two months late for his third Hepatitis B vaccine, will he have to start the course again?

No, there is no need to start the course again. The course should be completed with one further dose, and immunity checked two months later.

Q2.19 Are the two available commercial vaccines compatible during a course of immunization?

In the UK there are at present two commercial vaccines licensed. It is recommended that a course be completed with the same commercial vaccine.

Q2.20 What advice should be given to someone who fails to demonstrate immunity after a course of immunization?

The course should be repeated with the same commercial vaccine. If the individual fails to demonstrate immunity after the second course, a third course should be tried with a different commercial vaccine available in the UK. If the individual fails to develop immunity then, he/she is a non-responder and will need to take necessary precautions if exposed to hepatitis B, i.e. needle-stick injuries (see Q2.14).

Q2.21 What advice should be given for reducing HBV through sexual contact?

This is particularly relevant to people going abroad as there are many countries where the prevalence of HBV carriers is high (see Q2.2). Most of these carriers will otherwise be well. Risk can be reduced by avoiding or minimizing casual sex, and by the use of barrier methods of contraception, especially condoms.

Case history 1

A 29-year-old mother is concerned about the risk of Hepatitis B infection to herself and her 4-year-old daughter. She is also concerned about sending her daughter to the local nursery. Her 35-year-old husband has just come home after spending a week in hospital with arthritis and mild jaundice. The junior doctor confirmed just before discharge that microbiological tests had confirmed that her husband had suffered with acute Hepatitis B infection. What advice would you give to the mother?

Action

The husband is obviously infectious at the moment. It is also likely that he has been infectious for some weeks and may have passed on the infection to the wife if they have had unprotected sexual intercourse. The mother therefore needs to be informed of possible modes of transmission (see Q2.4). This may be a sensitive issue and needs to be handled with care.

At present it is not known how the husband may have acquired infection. It would be useful to test the mother's blood for indicators of Hepatitis B (see Box 2.2). If the results are negative, i.e. she is susceptible, an accelerated course of Hepatitis B vaccine should be recommended (See Q2.13, Q2.14). She should also be advised that until her husband is non-infectious they should use barrier methods of contraception during sexual intercourse. Serological testing would also identify whether the mother is an asymptomatic carrier and may have infected her husband. The daughter should also receive a course of Hepatitis B vaccination. There should be no reason why her daughter should not continue with her nursery education as normal.

Hepatitis C

Q2.22 What is Hepatitis C (HCV)?

There are a number of viruses that can cause hepatitis. Hepatitis C (HCV) is a blood-borne virus that was first identified in 1989. A diagnostic test became available in 1990 (see Q2.25).

Q2.23 How common is HCV?

Hepatitis C is a worldwide problem. The highest prevalence (more than 10 per cent) is in Egypt and other parts of Africa and South America; intermediate prevalence (2–10 per cent) includes Japan and parts of Southeast Asia; and low prevalence (less than 2 per cent) in the United Kingdom and United States. Current estimates of prevalence of HCV infection in the United Kingdom population are between 0.01 and 1 per cent (Foster et al., 1997).

Studies amongst blood donors in England estimated a prevalence of infection of 0.08–0.55 per cent (Ramsay et al., 1998). Between 1992 and 1996, laboratories in England and Wales reported 5,232 confirmed HCV infections (Ramsay et al., 1998). It is estimated that in the general population of the United Kingdom there may be 600,000 carriers (Waugh, 1998). To estimate the incidence and prevalence of HCV infection it is important to understand the significance of blood tests presently available (see Q2.25).

Q2.24 How is HCV transmitted?

Hepatitis C is a blood-borne virus and spreads by contact with blood or other body fluids from an infected person. Most commonly this is seen in those who use illegal drugs and share needles and infecting paraphernalia. HCV can also be transmitted through receipt of blood transfusions or clotting factor concentrate. In the United Kingdom all blood transfusions since September 1991 have been tested for HCV antibodies so that it can no longer spread in this way. Patients who may have received blood or blood products prior to September 1991 may have been exposed to HCV.

HCV can also spread via transplanted organs, tissues and bone grafts. Donors are therefore fully screened to minimize the risk. Mother-to-baby transmission can occur, but is uncommon. Sexual transmission has been reported although it does not seem to be easily transmitted by this route. There have been reports of infected surgeons passing the infection to their patients (Duckworth et al., 1999). In a substantial proportion of cases of acute HCV infection the mode of transmission of the virus is unclear.

Q2.25 What diagnostic tests are available for HCV infection?

A screening test for HCV became available in 1990. This test, which detects HCV antibodies, cannot distinguish between people who have been infected recently and those who were infected many years ago. A positive antibody test is evidence of previous exposure to HCV, but gives no indication of whether the virus is still present. This uncertainty can be resolved by a polymerase chain reaction test (Dore et al., 1997), which detects the presence of the virus itself rather than the antibody to HCV and can indicate persistent or chronic infection. In addition to these specific tests it is likely that levels of liver enzymes in the blood may be raised in patients with HCV infection.

Q2.26 What is the incubation period for HCV?

The incubation period is commonly between six and eight weeks (range two weeks to six months).

Q2.27 What are the symptoms of HCV?

The majority of people with HCV infection have no symptoms and they are often unaware they have the virus. Often the only evidence of infection is elevation of liver enzymes, which may lead to screening for HCV. Symptoms, when present, can be vague and can include a flu-like illness, sometimes with nausea and vomiting. Jaundice, which is a common sign of other forms of hepatitis, is unusual in HCV infection.

Q2.28 What is the natural history of infection with HCV?

Approximately 15–20 per cent of infected people get better completely. It is not known why some people are successful at fighting off the disease while others remain infected. A significant proportion (80–85 per cent) will develop chronic liver disease; some will progress to cirrhosis and liver cancer (Tong et al., 1995). Many people with HCV, however, may have normal liver function and it may take up to 20 years to develop serious liver disease.

Progression to chronic liver disease and cirrhosis is influenced by a number of factors (EASL, 1999):

- more rapidly progressive disease in people who acquire the infection at an older age;
- heavy consumption of alcohol;
- co-infection with another virus, HIV or Hepatitis B infection are important factors in progression of chronic hepatitis to cirrhosis.

Therefore those who inject drugs and have not had Hepatitis B should be strongly advised to consider Hepatitis A and B vaccination to prevent co-infection (see Q2.14, Q2.15, Q3.20).

Q2.29 Is there immunization for HCV?

At the present moment there is no vaccine available to prevent Hepatitis C.

Q2.30 Who is most at risk from HCV?

Individuals most at risk are those who come into contact with blood containing HCV. Currently it is not possible to find out who may be carrying the virus. Some patients may have been infected as a result of receiving contaminated blood before it was made safe in 1991 (see Q2.24). Intravenous drug users and those who participate in tattooing and body piercing are currently most at risk. A recent study on prevalence amongst two-thirds of the prison population in the Republic of Ireland reported one in three inmates infected with HCV, most probably related to intravenous drug use (Allwright et al., 1999). Anyone who works in an environment where blood might be easily transferred, i.e. healthcare staff, ambulance workers, firemen, police officers and prison workers, is at risk.

Q2.31 How long is a person infectious with HCV?

The natural history of HCV is not well understood. However, it is estimated that 85 per cent of individuals with acute infection will develop chronic disease (Waugh 1998). Infectivity depends on the amount of virus present in blood. Absence of HCV viraemia detectable by polymerase chain reaction indicates an extremely low risk of transmission (Dore et al., 1997) (see Q2.25).

Q2.32 What is the treatment of HCV?

Current treatment options have limited efficacy. Management of chronic HCV infection may depend on the severity of liver disease (see Q2.28). The main aim of treatment is to normalize liver function and to eliminate the virus from the blood during and after treatment. Not everyone with HCV infection is considered suitable for treatment and many patients may need only regular assessment to detect whether liver damage is occurring. The management of the patient would normally be shared by a specialist (liver unit) and the general practitioner. Until recently the only licensed treatment was interferon α. This drug has only limited efficacy and could give rise to a number of side-effects. The most recent promising development has been of ribavarin used in combination with interferon b. There are increasing reports that combination therapy with these two drugs is more effective than interferon α alone (McHutchinson et al., 1998).

The percentage of patients who have a sustained response to treatment is around 40 per cent. Response to treatment may depend on a number of factors, and a good response is seen in younger patients with mild disease and low viral load who have absence of cirrhosis or fibrosis (McHutchinson et al., 1998, Poynard et al., 1998).

Q2.33 Who should be screened for HCV?

Screening should only be undertaken following counselling, to ensure the patient gives informed consent for the procedure, as the treatment options are still limited (see Q2.32). Drug users who have shared any form of injecting equipment, including water, filters and spoons, and needles and syringes should be offered a test for HCV after counselling. Many are aware of the high incidence of HCV amongst this group, but a positive result can still be devastating to the individual.

Q2.34 How can HCV be prevented?

At the moment the prospects of HCV vaccine are remote and current treatment options are not very effective. The main elements of prevention and control of HCV would be to prevent further transmission. Blood for transfusions in the United Kingdom is screened for HCV and has been since 1991 (See Q2.24). Organ donors are also screened for HCV.

Appropriate infection control procedures in the healthcare setting also help to reduce transmission between patients and healthcare staff and vice versa (see Q1.14). There is an obvious need to provide education to those who are at the highest risk, in particular intravenous drug users (see Box 2.3). Safer sex messages and needle exchange schemes will also help to reduce the burden of disease.

Box 2.3 Prevention of HCV

Harm minimization for intravenous drug and/or cocaine users includes:

- Use only clean needles – do not share
- Disposing of needles safely – use a needle exchange scheme
- Do not share a toothbrush
- Do not share a razor
- Do not use a communal pot of water or other paraphernalia for injecting
- Do not share a rolled note for snorting cocaine
- Cover all cuts with a dressing

HCV is a fairly new disease and there is a lot to learn in the future. An appropriate information system should be established to track distribution of infection. Management of people who are already infected will also help to reduce transmission. Current treatment options should be regularly evaluated.

HIV and AIDS

Q2.35 What is AIDS?

Acquired immunodeficiency syndrome (AIDS) was first described in 1981 and represents the late clinical stage of infection with the human immunodeficiency virus (HIV). There are three stages of HIV infection: asymptomatic, symptomatic HIV-related disease, and AIDS.

Q2.36 How common is HIV/AIDS?

HIV transmission has been relentless since 1981 across all continents but especially throughout Africa, where 70 per cent of all HIV-infected people live (Piot et al., 2001). Latest estimates are that the cumulative total at the year 2000 was 56 million worldwide, 36 million of whom are still living with HIV (Piot et al., 2001).

In the United Kingdom by the end of September 2000 there were 43,026 reports of diagnosed HIV infections, 13,782 (32 per cent) of whom are known to have died (CDSC, 2000). In the United Kingdom there have been around 2,500 new cases of HIV infections diagnosed annually, however the last few years has shown an increasing trend. The infection is much more common in males than in females. The two commonest risk groups include homosexual men and those who inject drugs. The majority of cases are in those aged between 25 and 45 years.

Q2.37 How is HIV/AIDS transmitted?

The HIV is found in blood and body fluid. It can be transmitted via:

- sexual intercourse;
- percutaneous exposure to infected blood;
- from an infected mother to her child during birth (see Q2.46).

Q2.38 What is the incubation period?

The time taken from HIV exposure to the development of detectable antibodies is generally one to three months. The time from HIV infection to diagnosis of AIDS has a range of less than one year to 15 years or longer (Chin, 2000). Without effective anti-HIV therapy about half of infected adults will develop AIDS within 10 years.

Q2.39 How long is a person infectious?

Once the HIV infection is diagnosed the patient can pass on the virus throughout life.

Q2.40 What are the symptoms of HIV/AIDS?

After some weeks to months of exposure to HIV some patients develop a flu-like illness lasting for a week or two. Infected persons may then be free of clinical signs or symptoms for many months or years before other clinical manifestations develop. The HIV causes dysfunction of the immune system leading to opportunistic infections and several cancers. A case definition for AIDS was developed in 1987 and later revised in 1993 (see Box 2.4) and these diseases were accepted as meeting the definition of AIDS if other known causes of immunodeficiency had been ruled out.

Box 2.4 1987 CDC definition of AIDS in patients with laboratory evidence of HIV

A definite diagnosis of:

1. Bacterial infections, multiple or recurrent (any combination of at least two within a two-year period), in a child <13 years of age
2. Disseminated coccidioidomycosis
3. HIV encephalopathy (also termed 'HIV dementia', 'AIDS dementia' or 'subacute encephalitis caused by HIV')
4. Disseminated histoplasmosis
5. Isosporiasis with diarrhoea for > one month
6. Kaposi's sarcoma
7. Lymphoma of the brain (primary)
8. Non-Hodgkin's lymphoma of B cell or unknown immunological phenotype and one of the following histological types
   • Small non-cleaved lymphoma (Burkitt's or non-Burkitt's type)
   • Immunoblastic sarcoma (equivalent to any of the following, though not necessarily in combination – immunoblatic lymphoma, large-cell lymphoma, diffuse histiocytic lymphoma, diffuse undifferentiated lymphoma, high-grade lymphoma)

NB Lymphomas of T cell immunological phenotype, undescribed histological type, or 'lymphocytic', 'lymphoblastic', 'small cleaved' or 'plasmactyoid lymphocytic' type are not included here

9. Disseminated mycobacterial disease (other than Mycobacterium tuberculosis)
10. Extrapulmonary Mycobacterium tuberculosis involving at least one site outside the lungs
11. Recurrent Salmonella (non-typhoid) septicaemia
12. HIV wasting syndrome (emaciation, 'slim disease')

Or a presumptive diagnosis of:

1. Candidiasis of the oesophagus
2. Cytomegalovirus retinitis with loss of vision
3. Kaposi's sarcoma
4. Lymphoid interstitial pneumonia and/or pulmonary lymphoid hyperplasia in a child <13 years of age
5. Disseminated mycobacterial disease (acid-fast bacilli with species not identified by culture)
6. Pneumocystic carinii pneumonia
7. Toxoplasmosis of the brain in a patient > one month of age

The 1987 definition of AIDS was modified in 1992 by the addition of three clinical conditions in the presence of HIV infection: cervical cancer, two episodes of bacterial pneumonia in 12 months, and pulmonary tuberculosis

---

Q2.41 What is the natural history of AIDS?

Following infection, the time before onset of clinical disease varies from months to years. Although most patients initially have no characteristic symptoms, there is usually a gradual decline in immune function. In the 1980s and early 1990s virtually all patients who developed AIDS died in a few years. Since the introduction of effective highly active anti-retro-viral therapy (HAART) most patients are surviving much longer (Brettle, 2001) (see Q2.45). There is much to learn about the natural history of HIV as it has been known for only 20 years. With the availability of treatment and other effective measures to prevent infection, the epidemiology of HIV infection is constantly changing.

Q2.42 How is HIV/AIDS diagnosed?

The diagnosis of HIV infection may vary with presentation. A patient may present after being exposed to the infection, which can be confirmed by an HIV antibody test in the microbiology laboratory. Detectable antibodies may take between one and three months before the test is positive.

Another presentation could be via a variety of opportunistic infections or cancer without any definite history of exposure. An HIV antibody test will confirm the diagnosis. Further specialist tests include CD4 counts and viral load assays, which indicate seriousness of infection and are used to monitor disease and drug therapy (Zuckerman and Pillay, 2001).

Q2.43 Are patients ever tested without consent?

Patients are sometimes tested without consent but this should not occur, as a positive test may have a significant impact on these individuals and their families (see Q2.46, Q2.47, Q2.50).

Q2.44 Is there a vaccine to prevent HIV/AIDS?

No, there is at present no vaccine available. However, a number of trials are being conducted.

Q2.45 How is HIV treated?

HIV disease is caused by a virus entering human cells. There are at present no drugs that can completely cure HIV infection but there were a number of treatment developments in the mid-1990s that reduce viral load in a patient. The essence of drug therapy is to use agents in combinations that act at different phases of the virus life cycle. Present treatment includes a combination of the following three groups of drugs (Gazzard and Moyle, 1998):

1. nucleoside analogue reverse transcriptase inhibitors (NARTIs);
2. non-nucleoside reverse transcriptase inhibitors (NNRTIs);
3. protease inhibitors.

The treatment of HIV infection is undertaken by specialists in genito-urinary medicine clinics or infectious diseases units. Over and above drug therapy, medical and nursing support is necessary. With recent development in drug therapy, patients are living much longer and their quality of life has improved. However, a number of patients are unable to tolerate this therapy owing to side-effects, and compliance can be a problem. In addition, resistance is a problem common to all drugs used to treat HIV disease and monitoring is necessary (Zuckerman and Pillay, 2001).

Q2.46 How can HIV infection be prevented?

The most common transmission is through sexual intercourse. Measures to promote barrier methods of contraception, especially amongst gay men and those who travel abroad, is important. Blood for transfusion is now screened for HIV in the UK and is therefore safe. Other measures include education for those who inject drugs and the availability of a needle exchange schemes for those who continue to inject drugs, to prevent sharing of needles. Even sharing any paraphernalia can be a risk for viral infections to spread (see Q2.34).

Transmission from mother to baby can be reduced if the mother's HIV status is known, as early treatment can reduce the chance of developing infection. In the UK there is now a national programme for HIV screening during pregnancy (DoH, 1999a). As with all antenatal tests, this HIV screening is voluntary. Women are provided with information so that they may opt out if they wish.

Q2.47 What are other social issues important for patients with AIDS?

The diagnosis of HIV infection can have a devastating effect on a patient and his/her family. Confidentiality is of paramount importance. If a patient is undertaking a test for HIV this should be done only after counselling about the pros and cons of testing and the consequences of a positive test. Expert counsellors are available in genitourinary and family planning/sexual health clinics. Counselling will also be needed if a test is positive. Patients will also need support in the community and expert help should be sought from a clinical nurse specialist (HIV/AIDS). As patients are now living longer and their quality of life is improving they need advice on issues relating to social benefits, employment and life skills. Help should be available from social services. HIV infection can have a significant effect on the patient's family/carers, who will need appropriate support (see Box 2.5).

Box 2.5 Social and personal issues for patients with HIV/AIDS

- Social needs have increased since antiretroviral therapies

- People need considerable support with compliance issues and understanding that the medication has to be taken every day for life

- Psychological support is required because taking regular medication interferes with life and cannot always be taken privately, thus informing others that there is something wrong

- Financial problems are likely, because health improves and benefits are more difficult to obtain. Returning to work may be tiring, frequent hospital appointments and pill taking do not go down well with employers. Most people are reluctant to divulge their status, appear well and therefore employers think they are faking

- Availability of transport for hospital appointments is crucial as many patients do not drive and cannot afford taxi or public transport

- Concerns about travelling abroad may arise should the condition alter, and difficulty of explaining drugs to customs staff

- Pregnancy issues are now emerging as the heterosexual incidence increases. Young people in the main want children despite the risks, therefore support regarding the options is required

- GPs and practice nurses are still not recognizing the signs and symptoms, particularly in the younger age groups. Patients are therefore presenting in quite advanced stages of the virus

- A lot of support required for patients who have been on therapy for some time and are now experiencing some of the more unpleasant side-effects

- As younger people become infected, they need encouragement not to have body piercing and tattooing as this increases the risk of infecting others. It is common practice still for HIV-infected people to do this

- GPs and practice nurses need to understand that infected people need to be seen quickly or there needs to be discussion with a consultant if presenting with symptoms such as pyrexia, cough, ophthalmic or neurological symptoms

---

Q2.48 Can an HIV-infected mother breast feed a baby?

Breast feeding increases the risk of transmission of HIV from an infected mother to her baby. As nutritionally adequate and safe bottle feeding is available in the UK, breast feeding by HIV infected mothers is not recommended (DoH, 1999b).

Q2.49 What is the risk of transmission to a healthcare worker and vice versa?

There have been a number of documented cases of hepatitis B infection occurring in patients operated on by hepatitis B-infected surgeons. It is plausible that HIV, a blood-borne virus, could be transmitted under similar circumstances. However, experience to date is that the risk of transmission of HIV is considerably less as compared with hepatitis B – for example, from a needle stick injury (DoH, 1998c).

Q2.50 Is it true that life assurance premiums are increased for HIV-positive people?

If a patient has a life assurance policy then subsequent positive tests should not make any difference. However, if a patient has a positive test and seeks life assurance he or she is unlikely to get it.

Q2.51 Do some countries require mandatory HIV testing for tourists?

There are a few countries in the world that do require a certificate. As such requirements may change, tourists should enquire what certificates are necessary as and when they travel to a particular country. People should be referred to the genitourinary clinic for testing where possible, to avoid documentation on their medical records which may influence insurance policies at a later date.

Q2.52 Are special kits necessary for HIV testing, and if so, where are they obtained from?

No special kits are required for HIV testing. Clotted blood is sent to the local microbiological laboratory for testing. No tests should be undertaken without counselling and informed consent. People requesting a test should ideally be referred to the genitourinary clinic for counselling, testing and support.

Summary

Blood-borne diseases can be prevented by using barrier methods of contraception and safer injection techniques for drug users. Ideally, health promotion strategies will reduce the numbers of drug misusers but until this occurs users should be encouraged to reduce the risk of contracting one or more of these diseases. Healthcare staff should follow universal precautions at all times, and treat all patients as possible carriers of infection. Those at high risk should be offered Hepatitis B vaccine.

Chapter 3
Gastrointestinal infections

Introduction

The number of cases of food poisoning rose annually in England and Wales in the 10 years from 39,713 in 1988 to 93,932 in 1998 (Communicable Disease Surveillance Centre, Gastrointestinal Section, 1999). However, this is likely to be an underestimation of the actual numbers of cases. Some people who are infected may be asymptomatic or have very mild symptoms, whilst others who are ill may not seek medical help. Others may seek medical help but the infection may not be notified. Therefore the numbers of cases of food poisoning that are notified probably comprise the tip of the iceberg (see Figure 3.1).

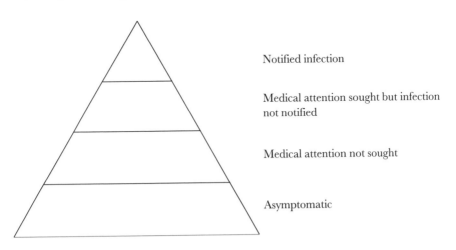

Notified infection

Medical attention sought but infection not notified

Medical attention not sought

Asymptomatic

Source: CDR Review 6:7 R93—R100 (1996).

Figure 3.1 The iceberg of gastrointestinal infections

Food poisoning is a major cause of morbidity amongst the population, and in some cases may cause death (Djuretic et al., 1996). As a community nurse, it is likely that you will be asked to treat and advise patients on what to do if they suspect that they have food poisoning or some other gastrointestinal infection, with regard to time off work and preventing the spread of infection to others in their household.

It is important that professional staff are clear about the definitions surrounding food poisoning so that the terminology, which can cause alarm, is used appropriately. The definitions are listed in Box 3.1.

Box 3.1 Definitions

Outbreak:
an incident in which two or more people, thought to have common exposure, experience a similar illness or proven infection.

Food-borne disease:
a disease of infectious or toxic nature caused or thought to be caused by the consumption of food or water.

Source: Evans et al. (1998).

Q 3.1 Which organisms cause food poisoning?

There are a number of organisms that can cause food poisoning and gastrointestinal infections. Table 3.1 lists the most common organisms that were responsible for outbreaks of gastrointestinal infectious disease in England and Wales in 1995 and 1996 (Wall et al., 1997).

Q 3.2 What procedure should be undertaken if food poisoning is suspected?

If a doctor suspects that a patient has food poisoning or a gastrointestinal infection then he or she should arrange for a stool specimen to be taken and tested at the local microbiology department. All positive results should be notified to the Consultant in Communicable Disease Control (CCDC) or Environmental Health Officer under the Public Health (Infectious Diseases) Regulation 1988. Official notification forms are available from the Environmental Health Department at the local council offices. All notifications are then forwarded to the Office of National Statistics for national surveillance purposes. At a local level, the CCDC will wish to monitor numbers of cases of food poisonings and, in conjunction with the local

Table 3.1 Common organisms responsible for outbreaks of infectious diseases

Organism	1995		1996	
	No. of outbreaks	No. of people affected*	No. of outbreaks	No. of people affected*
Small round structured virus (SRSV)	366	11 215	314	11 484
Salmonella species	120	2625	113	2321
Clostridium difficile	32	484	30	357
Clostridium perfringens	25	352	22	441
Rotavirus	23	383	31	483
Escherichia coli 0157	9	88	10	92
Scombrotoxin	9	54	6	23
Bacillus cereus	8	30	4	118
Campylobacter	4	140	8	99
Cryptosporidium	6	696	5	278
Astrovirus	1	10	9	218
Staphylococcus	1	7	5	146
B. subtilis	3	35	2	4
Shigella sonnei	-	-	4	51
Calcivirus	2	17	1	6
Other	9	279	7	101
Unknown	216	4470	163	3267
Total	834	20 885	734	19 489

*Note: Number of people affected is those with diarrhoea and/or vomiting +/- any other symptoms, not necessarily laboratory confirmed.
Source: Reproduced with kind permission from CDR.

Environmental Health Department, investigate suspected and confirmed outbreaks to protect the public's health from further occurrences. Food poisoning has always been of concern to the public, and attracts media attention. The *E. coli* 0157 outbreak in Scotland in 1996, when 18 people died and 496 cases of illness were reported, was linked to contaminated meat from a butcher's shop (Pennington, 1997) (see Q3.41–Q3.54). Investigations during and after that outbreak have had repercussions nationwide, and new guidelines have been implemented throughout the country in an attempt to prevent such an occurrence in the future.

Q3.3 What organisms are commonly responsible for food poisoning?

Various organisms can cause food poisoning and/or gastrointestinal spread, so the following sections look at some of these in more detail.

Table 3.2 lists clinical features of gastrointestinal infections, infestations and intoxications.

Table 3.2 Clinical features of gastrointestinal infections, infestations and intoxications

Causative agent	Incubation period	Common clinical features	Mode of transmission
Bacillus cereus emetic syndrome diarrhoeal syndrome	1–5 hours 8–16 hours	Nausea, vomiting Diarrhoea, abdominal pain	Ingestion of contaminated food
Campylobacter sp	1–11 days (usually 2–5 days)	Abdominal pain, profuse diarrhoea, malaise, vomiting is uncommon	Ingestion of contaminated food
Cholera	A few hours to 5 days (usually 2–3 days)	Profuse watery diarrhoea, rapid dehydration	Ingestion of contaminated food or water
Clostridium botulinum	8 hrs–8 days (usually 12–18 hours)	Dysphonia, diplopia, dysphagia, ptosis	Ingestion of contaminated food
Clostridium perfringens	8–22 hours (usually 12–18 hours)	Diarrhoea and abdominal pain	Ingestion of contaminated food
Cryptosporidium	2–5 days	Watery or mucoid diarrhoea	Faecal–oral, contaminated water, animal contact
Dysentery – amoebic	2–4 weeks	Bloody diarrhoea	Faecal–oral
Escherichia coli (VTEC)	1–6 days	Haemorrhagic colitis, haemolytic uraemic syndrome	Ingestion of contaminated food, faecal–oral
Giardia lamblia	5–25 days	Diarrhoea, abdominal cramps	Ingestion of contaminated food or water, faecal–oral
Hepatitis A	2–6 weeks	Fever, malaise, nausea, jaundice	Ingestion of contaminated food or water, faecal–oral
Salmonella typhi / paratyphi	1–3 weeks	Fever, malaise, nausea, constipation (early) diarrhoea (late)	Ingestion of contaminated food or water
Salmonellas	12–72 hours	Diarrhoea, vomiting and fever	Ingestion of contaminated food or water

Table 3.2 (contd)

Causative agent	Incubation period	Common clinical features	Mode of transmission
Shigella sp	1–7 days	Bloody diarrhoea *S. sonnei* generally mild, other species more severe	Faecal–oral, occasionally contaminated food or water
Staphylococcus aureus	1–7 hours (usually 2–4 hours)	Vomiting, abdominal pain	Ingestion of contaminated food
Viral gastroenteritis (rotavirus)	48 hours approx	Diarrhoea, vomiting	Faecal–oral
Viral gastroenteritis (small round structured virus)	24–48 hours	Diarrhoea, vomiting	Faecal–oral

Source: PHLS working party (1995a).

Q3.4 Are there any groups of people who are especially at risk of transmitting gastrointestinal infections?

Within the community there are groups of people who have greater potential to transmit gastrointestinal infections to others. There are national guidelines which recommend when these high-risk groups can resume normal work and leisure activities following gastrointestinal infection (Box 3.2).

Q3.5 What is the general infection control guidance for patients with gastrointestinal infections?

There are several important areas that must be addressed to control infection.

Hand washing

Thorough hand washing and drying is the most important factor in preventing the spread of diarrhoea and vomiting infections (see Table 3.2). This must be carried out by all carers attending to people who have symptoms, and also by patients themselves. Children should be supervised to ensure that they are washing their hands effectively.

Box 3.2 Groups 1–4 guidance on return to usual activities following gastro-intestinal illness <u>when organisms are not known</u>. For specific organisms see Q3.17, 3.38, 3.53, 3.69, 3.81, 3.97

Group 1	Food handlers	Can normally return to work once they have been symptom free for 48 hours. If in doubt seek advice from CCDC
Group 2	Healthcare, nursery and other staff who have contact with susceptible individuals	Can normally return to work once they have been symptom free for 48 hours. If in doubt seek advice from CCDC
Group 3	Children attending nurseries/playgroups and schoolchildren who cannot be relied on to maintain personal hygiene	Can normally return to nursery/school etc. once they have been symptom free for 48 hours. If in doubt seek advice from CCDC
Group 4	Infirm, disabled or elderly persons who are attending or residing in homes or other similar institutions	Can normally return to usual activities once they have been symptom free for 48 hours. If in doubt seek advice from CCDC

Source: PHLS Salmonella Working Party (1995a). Reproduced with kind permission from CDR.

- Hands should be washed after handling bedding, clothing or any equipment that has been in contact with the sick person.
- Hands should be washed before and after preparing or serving food.
- Patients and carers should wash hands after using the toilet.

Facilities

- Where possible the patient should use a toilet that has been designated specifically for that person.
- Soiled clothing and bed linen should be washed in a washing machine on a 'hot cycle'.

Environmental cleaning

It is recommended that either disposable or household gloves designated solely for the purpose of environmental cleaning are worn and that hands are washed and dried thoroughly after the procedure.

Ensure that the following areas are cleaned daily or when soiled using a soap solution (such as washing-up liquid and warm water) and disposable cloths. It is advisable to use a bleach spray in between thorough cleaning whilst the patient has symptoms, especially for:

- toilet seats;
- flush handles;

- wash hand basin taps;
- toilet door handles and/or pushes plates.

Hepatitis A

Q3.6 What is Hepatitis A (HAV)?

Hepatitis A (HAV), also known as infectious hepatitis, is a viral infection that causes inflammation of the liver and associated illness.

Q3.7 What causes HAV?

HAV is a non-enveloped virus, which survives acid conditions and resists the action of ether (Winter, 1999). It can survive for long periods in water or sewage.

Q3.8 How common is HAV?

Three patterns of disease have been identified (Chin, 2000):

1. sporadic cases (Maguire et al., 1995)
2. community-wide outbreaks due mainly to person-to-person transmission (Reintjes et al., 1999);
3. point source outbreaks related to contaminated food (Sundkvist et al., 2000).

The number of cases reported to the Public Health Laboratory Service (PHLS) has fallen over the past 10 years, although incidence does show a cyclical pattern (Maguire et al., 1992). The most recent peak was in 1990 (DoH, 1996a).

Improvements in hygiene and sanitation in developed countries have decreased transmission of the virus (see Figure 3.2). In England and Wales this trend has resulted in an increase in the proportion of susceptible adolescents and young adults (Gay et al., 1994).

HAV is associated with foreign travel and the prevalence of disease is higher outside the United Kingdom. The highest risk areas are Eastern Europe, the Indian sub-continent and the Far East. Of all cases reported to the PHLS in 1995, 13 per cent of patients revealed a history of foreign travel in the six weeks before they became ill (DoH, 1996a). A case control study in 1995 showed that the factors associated with increased risk of acquiring HAV included, apart from foreign travel, living with someone who has HAV and sharing a household with a child aged 3–10 years (Maguire et al., 1995).

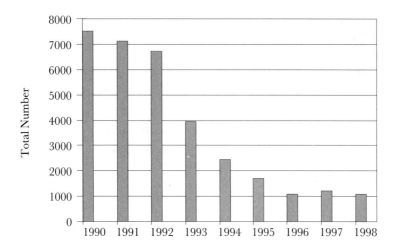

Figure 3.2 Hepatitis A Laboratory Reports – England and Wales, 1990–98.
Source: Communicable Disease Surveillance Centre: Gastrointestinal Section 2000.

Q3.9 What is the incubation period of HAV?

The incubation period is 15–50 days, with an average of 28–30 days
(Chin, 2000).

Q3.10 How is HAV transmitted?

HAV is transmitted through contaminated food or water and from person
to person via the faecal–oral route. An infected person is most infectious
approximately two weeks before the onset of symptoms, continuing for a
few days after the onset of jaundice (Chin, 2000).

Q3.11 Who is at risk of contracting HAV?

Any person not immune to the disease is at risk.

Q3.12 What are the signs and symptoms of HAV?

The signs and symptoms of infection with HAV are usually sudden in
their onset with:

•   anorexia;
•   nausea;

- abdominal discomfort;
- general malaise; followed by jaundice.

Clinical manifestations vary from a mild illness lasting 1–2 weeks to, rarely, a severe, disabling disease which may last several months. In many cases there are no signs and symptoms of illness at all – children are most likely to be asymptomatic. The severity of symptoms appears to increase with age. Adults are at increased risk of jaundice or more severe disease. HAV has not been reported to cause chronic infection (Teo, 1992).

Q3.13 How long do the symptoms last?

Usually 1–2 weeks.

Q3.14 Can HAV be caught twice?

No, previous infection provides immunity.

Q3.15 How is HAV diagnosed?

The signs and symptoms of infection with HAV cannot be distinguished clinically from other forms of hepatitis, and laboratory diagnosis is essential (Winter, 1999). The diagnosis of acute HAV is routinely based on the detection of anti-HAV Igm antibodies in serum during acute illness. Abnormalities of liver enzymes would also be present. A salivary test to detect antibodies is another method that has been used to screen travellers (Parry et al., 1987, Parry et al., 1988) and in outbreak investigations (Stuart et al., 1992).

Q3.16 How is it treated?

There is no specific treatment for HAV. Management mainly involves treatment of symptoms only.

Q3.17 Should a patient stay off work?

All cases including those in Risk Groups 1-4 (see Box 3.2) should be excluded from work, school or nursery for seven days after the onset of jaundice/other symptoms (Working Party of the PHLS Salmonella Committee, 1995).

Q3.18 Should symptomless contacts of a case of HAV stay off work?

No. Symptomless contacts of a case who are food handlers can continue food handling providing basic food hygiene precautions are observed (DoH, 1996b) (see Q3.5).

Q3.19 How is HAV prevented?

Hepatitis A infections are prevented by:

- ensuring safe water supplies and good food hygiene, with specific emphasis on hand washing (see Figure 1.1);
- sanitary disposal of faeces (Maguire et al., 1992) (see Box 1.1);
- vaccination of those who are at risk (see Q3.20);
- monitoring and surveillance of infection and follow-up of cases and their contacts (see Q3.2).

Apart from being immunized, travellers are advised to ensure good standards of food and personal hygiene to prevent infection. A booklet entitled *Health Advice for Travellers* (DoH 1999c), available at all Post Offices and helpful to all travellers, includes the recommendations listed in Box 3.3.

Box 3.3 Reducing the risk of Hepatitis A: recommendations for travellers

Always wash your hands after going to the lavatory, before handling food and before eating

If you have any doubt about the water available for drinking, washing food or cleaning teeth, boil it, sterilize it with disinfectant tablets or use bottled water – preferably carbonated with gas – in sealed containers

Avoid ice

It is usually safe to drink hot tea and coffee, wine, beer, carbonated water and soft drinks, and packaged or bottled fruit drinks

Eat freshly cooked food which is thoroughly cooked and still piping hot

Avoid food that has been kept warm

Avoid uncooked food unless you can peel or shell it yourself

Avoid food likely to have been exposed to flies

Avoid ice cream from unreliable sources, such as kiosks or itinerant traders

Avoid – or boil – unpasteurized milk

Uncooked shellfish, such as oysters, are a particular hazard

Source: DoH (1999c).

Q3.20 What immunization is available for HAV?

There are two types of immunization available, providing:

1. passive immunity;
2. active immunity (DOH. 1996a).

Passive immunity

Human normal immunoglobulin (HNIG) is recommended for those who have had recent, significant contact with a confirmed case of HAV. It provides rapid, short-lived protection against the infection if given at an early stage. In those who are incubating the infection it may reduce the severity of the infection.

Some religions do not accept human blood products; this must be considered to ensure informed consent for treatment is given (Tweed et al., 1999).

Active immunity

This is recommended for those who are identified as requiring long-term immunity, which includes:

- travellers to high-risk areas (see Q3.8);
- patients with chronic liver disease (see Q3.6);
- patients with haemophilia;
- occupational exposure, e.g. laboratory workers working directly with the virus;
- patients with HCV (see Q2.28);
- men who have sex with men.

Vaccination consists of a single dose (offering protection for one year) followed by a booster dose 6–12 months later (which increases protection to 10 years) (BNF, 2000).

Q3.21 Do close contacts of an infected individual need to be followed up?

Prophylaxis in the form of HNIG is recommended for household and close contacts of a case of HAV, although extending the contacts to recent household visitors and those who have eaten food prepared by the index case may be more effective in preventing further spread (DoH, 1996a).

Q3.22 What should happen if there is a suspected outbreak of HAV?

In circumstances where there are a number of linked cases of HAV the CCDC will advise on the measures necessary for control of the outbreak. In addition to advising on good hygiene, vaccination may be offered to the population deemed at risk: those who have been in close contact with the index cases (see Q3.20).

Q3.23 What are the implications for healthcare staff?

Healthcare staff should ensure that they follow the general infection control practices with all patients and take precautions when handling faeces.

If the healthcare worker has the infection he or she should remain off work for seven days after the onset of jaundice (see Q3.17).

Q3.24 Are nursery nurses classed as an at-risk group for HAV?

Yes (see Box 3.2).

Q3.25 Is active immunization recommended for child travellers?

Yes.

Q3.26 If a patient is late coming for his booster Hep A vaccination, should he have a blood test to check his immunity?

There is no need to test for immunity – the course should be repeated.

Q3.27 Should patients routinely have a blood test to check Hep A status prior to a course of vaccination?

There is no need to check Hepatitis A status before immunization.

Case history 2

A patient is due to work in Israel for one year and is concerned, among other things, about acquiring hepatitis A infection. He will be living in first-class accommodation but will not be catering for himself.

Action

Although Israel has implemented a universal hepatitis A immunization campaign (Meheus, 1999) visitors to the country are advised to have vaccination against HAV to provide protection. The vaccine is 88 per cent effective after two weeks and 99 per cent effective after four weeks. However, it is still recommended that travellers also take basic precautions to reduce the risk of exposure to this and other viruses. The patient should be advised to follow the advice set out in the Health Advice to Travellers booklet (see Q3.19, Box 3.3).

Box 3.4 Basic food hygiene

Buying food
- Check the use by/sell by date
- Take a coolbox/insulated bag with you when you shop in hot weather; buy perishable foods at the end of your shopping
- Buy smaller quantities more often to ensure freshness
- Take chilled and frozen food home quickly and put it in your fridge or freezer at once

Storing food
- Clean and defrost your fridge regularly
- Store raw and cooked food separately. Keep raw meat and fish in covered containers in the bottom of your fridge to avoid blood dripping on to other foods
- When unpacking shopping put new food supplies at the back of the cupboard so that you rotate your food supply and use by the recommended date

Preparing food
- Wash your hands before handling food and after handling raw meat and fish
- Keep cooked and uncooked foods separate and if possible keep a separate chopping board for meat
- Defrost meat, poultry and fish thoroughly before cooking
- Keep dogs and cats out of the kitchen when you are preparing food

Cooking
- Ensure meat is cooked evenly throughout
- Reheated food should be heated to a temperature of no less than 75°C, i.e. piping hot

Serving food
- Cooked food should be eaten immediately or cooled rapidly before refrigeration or freezing
- Warm food provides an ideal environment for bacteria to multiply so it must be kept above 63° or below 5°C

Cleaning the kitchen
- Wash worktops and utensils between cooked and uncooked foods
- Wipe up spills on work surfaces and the floor as soon as possible
- Try to keep separate cloths for different cleaning tasks and disinfect them regularly

General
- Keep pet feeding bowls separate from family dishes

Cryptosporidiosis

Q3.28 What is cryptosporidiosis?

Cryptosporidium is a parasitic protozoan organism that causes gastro-intestinal infection if it is ingested as a cyst. Cryptosporidiosis is an infection caused by *Cryptosporidium*. The infective dose is thought to be quite low. In those who are immuno-compromised the illness may be much longer and serious disease may result (see Q3.34).

Q3.29 Where is cryptosporidium found?

It is found in the gastrointestinal tract of man and farm animals and in water that has been contaminated with infected faeces.

Q3.30 How common is cryptosporidiosis?

Cryptosporodiosis is a relatively common disease and accounts for approximately 4000–5000 notifications each year (Figure 3.3). The majority of cases are sporadic, although the organism can cause outbreaks of infection.

Between 1988 and 1998 *Cryptosporidium* was associated with 25 outbreaks of infection traced to public water supplies and swimming pools (Furtado et al., 1998) (Figure 3.4). However, most outbreaks occurred in situations where oocysts were not detected in water supplies (Bouchier, 1998).

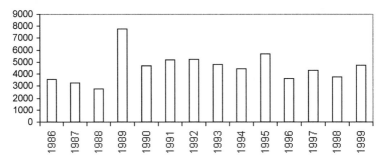

Figure 3.3 Cryptosporidium Laboratory Reports England and Wales, all identifications, 1986–99. Source: Communicable Disease Surveillance Centre: Gastrointestinal Section 2000.

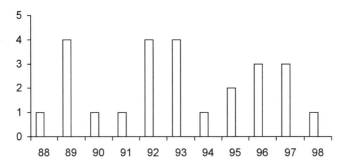

Figure 3.4 UK outbreaks of Cryptosporidiosis associated with public water supplies 1988–98. Source: Furtado et al., 1998.

Q 3.31 How is cryptosporidiosis transmitted?

It can be transmitted from domestic and farm animals, via contaminated water, food and from an infected person (PHLS Salmonella Committee, 1995a).

Q3.32 Who is susceptible?

Anyone ingesting the oocyst is vulnerable although those who are immuno-compromised are particularly susceptible and excrete large numbers of the organism if infected. Staff and children in nurseries and families who are in contact with an infected person are also particularly vulnerable (PHLS Salmonella Committee, 1995a). Previous infection does not provide immunity.

Q3.33 What is the incubation period?

This is between 2 and 14 days.

Q3.34 What are the signs and symptoms?

The illness is characterized by very watery diarrhoea which, although generally self-limiting, can last up to two to three weeks (Bouchier, 1998). The signs and symptoms of cryptosporidiosis are:

- watery diarrhoea with abdominal cramps;
- weight loss;
- anorexia;
- flatulence;
- malaise;
- nausea, vomiting, fever and myalgia may also be experienced.

Some patients may also report increased abdominal cramps and diarrhoea immediately after eating (Mandell et al., 1990; Chin 2000). However, it is also possible for people to be infected but be asymptomatic. In patients who are immuno-compromised, symptoms may be particularly severe as they may be unable to clear the parasite, which may then contribute to the patient's death (Chin, 2000).

Q3.35 How is it diagnosed?

Stool samples are tested in the microbiology laboratory for the presence of oocysts.

Q3.36 Can the stool sample be stored overnight before transportation to the laboratory?

Yes. The sample can be stored overnight, in a designated fridge for specimens. The sample should be clearly labelled with the name and date of birth of the patient and the time and date the specimen was taken. It is important that the accompanying request form is completed, including clinical details of the patient and recent antimicrobial therapy. The specimen should be transported in a leak-proof container and staff should be aware of how to clean up spillages quickly and safely (see Box 1.1).

Q3.37 Can patients be treated for cryptosporidiosis?

There is currently no recognized specific treatment for cryptosporidiosis except for treatment of the symptoms. In cases where the symptoms are severe patients may need to be hospitalized for fluid and electrolyte replacement.

Q3.38 Should a patient stay off work?

The general rule is that anyone reporting a gastrointestinal infection should stay off work until he or she has been symptom free for 48 hours (see Q3.4, Box 3.2 for exclusion of food handlers and high-risk groups).

Infected people may continue to excrete the organism for up to two weeks after they are clinically well, therefore patients should be reminded about the importance of personal hygiene, in particular hand washing.

Q3.39 How is it prevented?

Prevention of person-to-person spread

Patients with cryptosporidiosis should be advised on personal hygiene and hand washing (see Q3.5).

Surveillance

Confirmed cases of cryptosporidiosis are investigated by the local environmental health officer (see Q3.2). Most cases are sporadic, some associated with outbreaks. If an outbreak is suspected (more than one linked case) then the Consultant in Communicable Disease Control should be informed and an outbreak team instigated.

Monitoring

Public water supplies are maintained to prevent the water becoming contaminated and are monitored regularly to ensure that the water is fit to drink (Bouchier, 1998). It is possible for *Cryptosporidium* to be present in source water and it is therefore the water company's job to reduce the risk of oocysts being present in tap water. However, *Cryptosporidium* is known to be resistant to chlorine and so the water companies have to rely on other methods, such as filtration, to reduce the numbers of oocysts that may be present. Immuno-compromised patients are therefore advised to *boil all water* prior to consumption to prevent potential infection from the water by *Cryptosporidium* oocysts (see Q3.32, Q3.34).

Q3.40 Are there any specific infection control precautions required?

Clinical staff should take the usual infection control precautions when handling any blood or body fluids, i.e. wearing a plastic apron and a pair of gloves and washing hands thoroughly when the procedure is complete. The patient must be encouraged to be scrupulous with personal hygiene and hand washing after using the lavatory and before preparing/eating food to prevent further spread within his or her home (see Q3.5).

Case history 3

A 25-year-old male attended the surgery reporting a three-day history of abdominal cramps and severe watery diarrhoea. It appears that he went windsurfing in a river two days before the onset of symptoms and at one stage fell into the water, swallowing a large amount. He still has watery diarrhoea and is feeling extremely unwell. He is, however, keen to get back to work in the local hotel kitchens as soon as possible because he is short of money and if he doesn't work he doesn't get paid.

Action

The practice nurse should arrange for a stool specimen to be sent to the microbiology laboratory for identification of the causative organism. In the meantime the patient can be reassured that whilst waiting for the results from the laboratory he can be helped to manage his symptoms. The patient should be encouraged not to return to work without the agreement of the local environmental health department. The nurse can help the patient by informing the Consultant in Communicable Disease Control that the chef has a gastrointestinal infection so that consideration can be given as to whether formal exclusion is necessary. Formal exclusion would entitle the chef to continue to be paid whilst he remained away from work. For further information, help, advice or leaflets the practice nurse should contact the infection control nurse working with the Consultant in Communicable Disease Control.

E. coli 0157 infection

Q 3.41 What is *E. coli* 0157?

Escherichia coli (*E. coli*) is a gram-negative bacterium and is part of normal bowel flora. It is a major cause of urinary tract infections, mainly because of the proximity of the bowel to the urethra, and was found to be responsible for 26 per cent of hospital acquired infections, mostly of the urinary tract (Meers et al., 1981). It is important that community nurses are able to explain the difference to a client between *E. coli* infection and one caused by *E. coli* 0157.

Escherichia coli 0157 (*E. coli* 0157) is a verocytotoxin-producing *Escherichia coli* (VTEC). It is pathogenic, which means that it can cause disease in man, by producing toxins that can cause illness. *E. coli* 0157 is the most common VTEC responsible for human infection in the United Kingdom (PHLS, 2000a).

E. coli 0157 has been found to grow optimally at a temperature of 37° C and the majority of outbreaks occur in the summer months (PHLS, 2000a; Wall et al., 1996).

Q3.42 How common is *E. coli* 0157?

E. coli 0157 was first discovered in 1982 (Wall et al., 1996). Most cases in England and Wales (80 per cent) appear to be sporadic. Total notifications have been steadily rising since 1992 (PHLS) (see Figure 3.5).

Q3.43 What is the incubation period for *E. coli* 0157?

The incubation period is one to six days, with a reported range of one to 14 days (PHLS, 1995b).

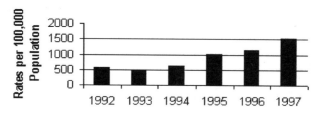

Figure 3.5 *E. coli* 0157 isolated in the United Kingdom: 1992–97. Source: Communicable Disease Surveillance Centre: Gastrointestinal Section 2000.

Q3.44 How is *E. coli* 0157 transmitted?

Dairy and beef cattle are a reservoir for *E. coli* 0157 although other farm animals have been implicated (PHLS, 2000a). It has been shown to be transmitted via food and water to humans, and from person to person (Stevenson and Hanson, 1996).

Q3.45 Who is at risk of contracting *E. coli* 0157?

The infectious dose appears to be low. The highest incidence of diagnosed *E. coli* 0157 infection is in children under 5 years of age (PHLS, 1995b).

Q3.46 What are the signs and symptoms of *E. coli* 0157?

Symptoms vary from mild and non-bloody diarrhoea to haemorrhagic colitis and severe abdominal pain with bloody diarrhoea. The lack of pyrexia can help in distinguishing this infection from other bacterial gastrointestinal infections such as shigella. In some cases the infection may lead to complications such as haemolytic uraemic syndrome (HUS) (see Q3.55).

Q3.47 How long do the symptoms last?

In uncomplicated infections symptoms are usually self-limiting, lasting approximately eight days.

Q3.48 Can the infection be caught twice?

Yes. Previous infection does not provide immunity and there is no vaccine.

Q3.49 How is it diagnosed?

Infection is diagnosed by culture of *E. coli* 0157 in faeces. All stool specimens are now routinely tested for *E. coli* 0157. Isolation from faeces is routinely successful only if samples are obtained within four days of the onset of symptoms (Stevenson and Hanson, 1996).

Q3.50 How is *E. coli* 0157 treated?

The value of antibiotics in the management of a straightforward infection with *E. coli* 0157 without complications and the duration of faecal excretion of the organism have not been established (Stevenson and Hanson, 1996; PHLS, 2000a). Anti-motility agents are not recommended for

patients, particularly children, who are suspected of having infection with
E. coli 0157. Studies have found that patients who develop HUS are more
likely to have had anti-motility drugs (Mead and Griffin, 1998).

Q3.51 How is *E. coli* 0157 prevented?

Prevention relies on:

- good hygiene by the general population in their personal lives;
- high standards of hygiene in retail establishments, on farms etc. to
  prevent the spread of the disease and consequential contamination of
  foodstuffs meant for human consumption;
- thorough cooking of meat – *E. coli* 0157 is destroyed by cooking at 70°C;
- guidance on hygiene in schools and nurseries and when on farm visits;
- prompt reporting of suspected or confirmed cases so that investigation
  can take place and further cases be prevented (see Q3.2).

The community nurse should advise the patient to follow the general
infection control guidance for patients with gastrointestinal infection to
prevent spread to family and friends (see Q3.5).

Q3.52 What are the implications for community staff?

If healthcare staff are seeing a patient with *E. coli* 0157 infection they
should follow general infection control guidelines and take precautions
when handling faeces (see Q3.5, Box 1.1).

Q3.53 When can the patient return to work/school/nursery?

In general, all those in risk groups 1–4 (see Box 3.2) should be excluded
until two consecutive negative faecal specimens, taken after recovery and
at least 48 hours apart, have been obtained (PHLS, 2000a).

Q3.54 What advice should be given to contacts of a case of *E. coli* 0157?

Cross-infection within the household has been well documented. All
contacts should be advised of general hygiene precautions that they can
take (see Q3.2).

Household contacts of a case who are in risk groups 1–4 (see Box 3.2)
should be excluded until two consecutive negative faecal specimens have
been obtained (PHLS, 2000a).

Household contacts who are not in risk groups 1–4 do not need to routinely submit faeces for examination, although for the purposes of surveillance and investigation they may sometimes be asked to do so by Public or Environmental Health Departments.

Q3.55 What is HUS?

Haemolytic uraemic syndrome (HUS) develops in about 6 per cent of patients, usually two to 14 days after the onset of diarrhoea, and is the most common cause of acute renal failure in children (Boyce et al., 1995). Other symptoms may include anuria and neurological complications such as seizures, coma and hemiparesis.

It is a more common complication in young children and the elderly and has a case fatality rate of approximately three to five per cent (Wall et al., 1996). A small percentage of those surviving may have long-term renal impairment or neurological damage as a result of the infection (Boyce et al., 1995).

Case history 4

You are called by a mother of a 3-year-old toddler who attends a local nursery. She has been informed that two children from the nursery have been diagnosed as having E. coli 0157 infection and one is in hospital very poorly. She is understandably very concerned and wants further information.

Action

The mother should be advised concerning signs and symptoms (see Q3.46) and on good hygiene within the home (see Q3.5).

In addition, this infection is of major public health importance, therefore it is wise to contact the local public health department, assuming that they have not been in contact with you, to seek further advice and to ensure that appropriate surveillance and follow-up are being done within the community.

Campylobacter infection

Q3.56 What is campylobacter infection?

Camplyobacter is a gastrointestinal infection associated with diarrhoea, malaise, fever and abdominal pain. The stools may be very watery or grossly bloodstained (see Q3.62).

Q3.57 What causes camplyobacter?

Campylobacter is a gram-negative bacterium that can cause gastrointestinal infection. Since 1981 campylobacter has been the most common enteric pathogen isolated from humans, although it is less well known than some gastrointestinal infections such as salmonella (Pebody et al., 1997).

There are a number of different campylobacters. *Campylobacter jejuni* and (rarely) *Campylobacter coli* are the usual causes of infection in humans.

Q3.58 How common is camplyobacter?

Campylobacter was first identified in 1977 as an important human pathogen and is now the leading cause of infective diarrhoea in England and Wales (Skirrow, 1977; Djuretic et al., 1996). Common source outbreaks have been reported most often associated with poultry, unpasteurized milk and contaminated water (Pebody et al., 1997) (see Q3.60; Figure 3.6 demonstrates the increasing incidence).

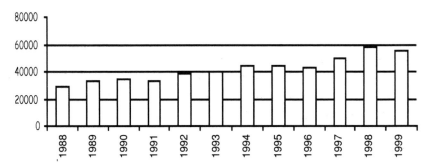

Figure 3.6 Campylobacter: laboratory reports to CDSC – Faecal isolates in England and Wales 1988–99. Source: Communicable Disease Surveillance Centre: Gastrointestinal Section 2000.

It is probable that there is a huge under-reporting of this infection. A community survey carried out in 1982 suggested that there might be as many as 500,000 cases of campylobacter infection each year (Kendall and Tanner, 1982). It is unlikely that these figures will have altered much. The reasons for under-reporting may be the fact that a number of people never seek medical advice because the symptoms are not severe enough or do not last long enough for the patient to seek medical help, or that it is not reported by the diagnosing doctor (see notification of suspected food poisoning, Figure 3.1).

Q3.59 What is the incubation period for campylobacter?

The incubation period is 1–10 days, but is usually 2–5 days (Chin, 2000).

Q3.60 How is campylobacter transmitted?

It has been associated with consumption of contaminated food such as undercooked poultry, contaminated water, inadequately pasteurized or raw milk, and contact with infected pets such as puppies and kittens. It is also suspected that the organism can be transferred to pasteurized milk from birds who peck milk-bottle tops (Hudson et al., 1991). Person-to-person spread is rare (Donaldson and Donaldson, 2000).

Q3.61 Who is at risk?

Anyone who eats contaminated food, or drinks contaminated fluids such as milk.

Q3.62 What are the signs and symptoms of campylobacter?

There may be a 24-hour period of fever and malaise, and aching limbs and backache prior to the onset of diarrhoea. In some people the onset of diarrhoea is very sudden and explosive accompanied by abdominal pain, profuse, offensive-smelling, bile or bloodstained diarrhoea and malaise. Vomiting is uncommon (Skirrow, 1977).

Q3.63 How long do the symptoms last?

Gastrointestinal infection with campylobacter is usually a self-limiting disease which lasts on average about a week and no longer than 10 days (Chin, 2000).

Q3.64 Can campylobacter infection be caught twice?

Yes. Previous infection does not confer immunity.

Q3.65 How is it diagnosed?

Diagnosis is made by isolating the organism in faecal samples. It takes the microbiology laboratory about 24 to 48 hours to culture the sample.

Q3.66 How is campylobacter treated?

Symptoms should be treated to prevent dehydration, e.g. fluid and electrolyte replacement. Anti-microbials are not normally necessary but antibiotics such as ciprofloxacin or erythromycin can be prescribed in cases where symptoms are severe or prolonged (BNF, 2000).

Q3.67 How long is a person infectious?

An infected person can continue to excrete the organism in his or her faeces for several weeks following infection. However, once the stools are formed and symptoms have subsided, providing the person observes a good standard of hygiene the risk is limited.

Q3.68 How is campylobacter prevented?

Campylobacter infections are prevented through observing basic food hygiene principles (see Box 3.4).

The community nurse should advise the patient to follow the general infection control guidance for patients with gastrointestinal infection to prevent spread to family and friends (see Figure 1.1, Q3.5).

Q3.69 What are the implications for healthcare staff?

If healthcare staff are looking after a patient with campylobacter infection they should follow general infection control guidelines and take precautions when handling faeces (see Box 1.1, Q3.5).

If the healthcare worker has the infection he or she should remain off work until he or she has been symptom free for 48 hours (see Box 3.2).

Case history 5

Over the course of a couple of days it comes to the practice nurse's attention that there has been an increased number of people arriving at the surgery complaining of gastrointestinal infection. The GP has arranged for some stool specimens to be collected and tested. It appears that the patients had all attended a barbecue at a local school fête.

Action

The practice nurse should inform the infection control nurse / CCDC so that investigation can be started in conjunction with the Environmental Health Department. (see Q3.2). The nurse should provide information to the cases and their families with regard to good personal hygiene and when they can return to work or school (see Q3.5, Box 3.2).

Salmonella infection

Q3.70 What is salmonella infection?

Salmonella is an important cause of gastrointestinal infection in humans. It is usually a self-limiting infection and the main objective of treatment is to prevent dehydration, particularly in the elderly and the very young (see Q3.80).

Rarely, salmonellosis can lead to bacteraemia and may also in a small percentage of cases cause widespread or local infections such as abscesses (soft tissue, hepatic or splenic), meningitis, endocarditis, arteritis or arthritis (Chin, 2000) (see Q3.73).

Q3.71 What causes salmonella infection?

Salmonella are non-sporing gram negative rods (Mandell et al., 1990). Salmonella have been isolated from almost all animal species including pigs, cows, domestic animals, poultry and reptiles, who may carry the organisms without showing clinical signs of infection (Ward, 2000; CDR, 2000a, 2000b), although the media portray this as a chicken and egg infection.

Q3.72 Who is at risk?

Anyone who ingests the bacteria is at risk. However, the young, elderly and immunosuppressed are most vulnerable.

Q3.73 What are the signs and symptoms of salmonella?

There is a sudden onset of:

- abdominal pain;
- diarrhoea;
- headache;
- nausea;
- vomiting (occasionally);
- a high temperature is almost always present.

Very occasionally the infection may develop into septicaemia or localize in any tissue of the body, producing widespread or local infections such as abscesses (soft tissue, hepatic or splenic), meningitis, endocarditis, arteritis or arthritis (Chin, 2000).

Q3.74 What is the incubation period?

The incubation period is from six to72 hours, but most commonly 12–36 hours.

Q3.75 How long do the symptoms last?

Symptoms may last several days, although excretion of the organism may last several weeks after the symptoms have subsided. In a few cases a carrier state may persist for several months (Chin, 2000).

Q3.76 How common is salmonella infection?

Although salmonella is probably one of the best known organisms to cause food poisoning it is less common than campylobacter (see Q3.56–Q3.69). There are different types of salmonella. The most common in England and Wales are *Salmonella enteritidis* and *Salmonella typhimurium*. Salmonellosis is more prevalent in the summer months.

Figure 3.7 shows the numbers of cases notified to the Communicable Disease Surveillance Centre for England and Wales between 1981 and 1999. It can be seen that although there was a steady rise in the numbers of cases during the 1990s, the numbers are now declining. It is suggested that this change may be due to improvements in food hygiene and vaccination of poultry flocks (CDR, 2000b).

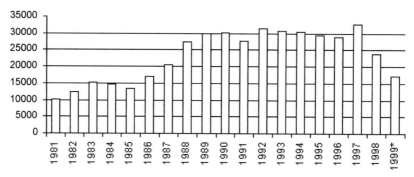

Figure 3.7 Salmonella in humans: faecal and unknown reports excluding S. typhi & S. paratyphi, England and Wales, 1981–99. *Provisional data. Source: PHLS, Laboratory of Enteric Pathogens; PHLS Salmonella data set.

Q3.77 How is salmonella transmitted?

Salmonella infection is passed by ingestion of the bacteria. This may occur in any of the following ways:

• inadequate cooking of raw meat, especially poultry;
• eating undercooked eggs;

- poor hygiene following contact with wild or domestic animals enabling spread via faecal–oral route (see Q3.71);
- poor hygiene following contact with infected person or carrier enabling spread via the faecal–oral route;
- poor hygiene in the kitchen allowing raw meat to contaminate cooked meat/salad foods (see Box 3.4);
- inadequate pasteurization of milk.

Salmonella has been responsible for many food poisoning outbreaks, accounting for 32 per cent of all outbreaks in England and Wales from 1992 to 1994 (Djuretic et al., 1996).

Q3.78 Can the infection be caught twice?

Yes, previous infection does not provide immunity.

Q3.79 How is salmonella diagnosed?

The infection is diagnosed by clinical history and positive microbiology. Stool samples should be sent to the microbiology laboratory for isolation and culture, which takes about 24 to 48 hours. Salmonella is routinely looked for in all stool specimens.

Q3.80 How is salmonella treated?

Symptoms should be treated to prevent dehydration. Occasionally hospitalization is necessary for replacement of fluids and electrolytes. Antibiotics are rarely prescribed because the infection tends to be short lived and antibiotics may extend the length of time a person may excrete the organism (Chin, 2000). However, where symptoms are severe or invasive, patients may be treated with ciprofloxacin (BNF, 2000).

Q3.81 Should a patient stay off work?

The general rule is that anyone reporting a gastrointestinal infection should stay off work, or school, until they have been symptom free for 48 hours.

Q3.82 How is it prevented?

Salmonella infections are prevented through observing basic food hygiene principles (see Box 3.4), such as storage of raw meat, hand washing, cooking eggs and meat thoroughly, pasteurization of milk and correct processing of drinking water. Caterers are requested not to use uncooked raw eggs in any meal they supply to the public but to use pasteurized eggs instead (Ejidokum et al., 2000; Sin et al., 2000).

The community nurse should advise the patient to follow the general infection control guidance for patients with gastrointestinal infection to prevent spread to family and friends (see Box 3.5).

Q3.83 What are the implications for healthcare staff?

If healthcare staff are looking after a patient with salmonella infection they should follow general infection control guidelines and take precautions when handling faeces (see Box 1.1).

If a healthcare worker has the infection he or she should remain off work until he or she has been symptom free for 48 hours.

Case history 6

A 6-month-old baby is confirmed as having salmonella infection from a stool sample. The baby has had symptoms for over a week and is beginning to get better. The child has not had antibiotics but care has been taken to ensure that fluid levels are maintained. There are no other members of the child's family with symptoms. The child attends nursery three mornings a week and the nursery has contacted the health visitor because the staff want to know whether they can accept the child back in the nursery yet or not.

Action

The child is in Risk Group 3 (see Box 3.2) and the key requirements are that the baby has been symptom free for at least 48 hours prior to returning to the nursery, and that the nursery can be relied on to carry out a high standard of infection control with regard to handling dirty nappies, hand washing and food hygiene.

Shigellosis (bacterial dysentery)

Q3.84 What is shigellosis?

Shigellosis is a gastrointestinal infection characterized by diarrhoea, abdominal cramps, bloody and mucousy stools and pyrexia (see Q3.90). It is very infectious. The infectious dose is very low, with only 10–100 organisms found to cause clinical infection in volunteers (Chin, 2000), and it has been found to be the causative organism for many outbreaks in the community.

Q3.85 What causes it?

It is caused by a type of bacteria called *Shigella*. The most prevalent of this species in the United Kingdom is *Shigella sonnei*, which accounts for 94 per cent of all *Shigella* isolates (Crowley et al., 1997). Other species that are not indigenous include *Shigella boydi*, *Shigella dysenteriae* and *Shigella flexneri* (Newman, 1993).

Q3.86 How common is it?

Shigella infection is highly communicable. It is most prevalent amongst pre-school and nursery children and it is responsible for a number of community-based outbreaks each year. A study of outbreaks of gastro-intestinal infection in schools in England and Wales between 1992 and 1994 showed that *Shigella sonnei* infection was responsible for 18 per cent of all such outbreaks (Evans and Maguire, 1996) (see Figure 3.8).

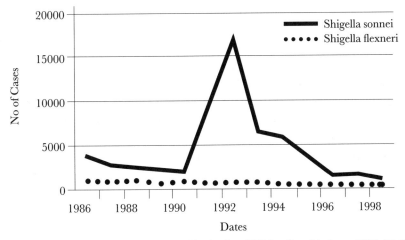

Figure 3.8 Shigella laboratory reports: England and Wales, faecal isolates, 1986–98. Source: Communicable Disease Surveillance Centre: Gastrointestinal Section 2000.

Q3.87 What is the incubation period?

Twelve to 96 hours, but usually one to three days.

Q3.88 How is it transmitted?

Shigella species are spread from person to person via the faecal–oral route. There are a number of recorded outbreaks describing transmission either within a family (Old et al., 2000); associated with eating canteen food (Maguire et al., 1998) or associated with hotels and restaurants (McDonnell et al., 1995); in child day-care centres (Mohle-Boetani et al., 1995); and via contaminated tap handles (Hospital Infection Control, 1996).

Because the infective dose is small it can be passed quickly between people on hands without having to multiply on food first, as with other infections such as salmonella.

Q3.89 Who is at risk?

Everybody coming in contact with the organism is susceptible. Previous infection with the organism confers no long-lasting protection against further infection (Newman, 1993). Breastfeeding has been found to be protective for the infant (Chin, 2000).

Q3.90 What are the signs and symptoms?

Most people with signs and symptoms of shigellosis will complain of diarrhoea and many will have associated stomach cramps, pyrexia, nausea and vomiting. The presence of blood and mucous in the stools is not uncommon. The disease is usually more severe in children than adults (Chin, 2000). *Shigella sonnei* is usually a mild infection and the acute symptoms will have subsided after 24 hours, although loose stools may continue for another few days (Newman, 1993).

Asymptomatic infection within households where other members of the family are symptomatic has been reported to range from 8 to 20 per cent (Chin, 2000).

Q3.91 How long do the symptoms last?

Although the infection is usually self-limiting, the symptoms may last from four to seven days (Chin, 2000).

Q3.92 Can the infection be caught twice?

Yes.

Q3.93 How is it diagnosed?

Diagnosis is made by clinical history and positive microbiology from a stool sample. Laboratory results usually take about 24 hours to report.

Q3.94 How is it treated?

Symptoms should be treated to prevent dehydration, using fluid and electrolyte replacement. Antibiotics are not generally indicated in mild cases of the infection (BNF, 2000). The selective use of antibiotics may, however, be indicated if the disease is severe or to protect contacts, particularly in an outbreak (Newman, 1993).

Q3.95 How is it prevented?

Good sanitation and hygiene facilities as well as hygienic practices should limit the risk of person-to-person spread.

The revised guidelines for the control of *Shigella sonnei* infection and other infective diarrhoeas identify the following as important measures to be taken within schools and nurseries (PHLS Working Group on the control of *Shigella sonnei* infection, 1993):

- Adequate toilet facilities including toilet paper, soap warm water and paper towels.
- Supervised hand washing in nurseries and infant schools, after using the toilet and before mealtimes.
- Written regimes for thorough cleaning of toilets and changing areas; disinfection of toys and equipment.
- Exclusion from nursery and school of children with diarrhoeal illness until symptom free and with formed stool.
- Hygiene advice to be offered to contacts of symptomatic individuals.
- Safe working practices by staff when changing children's nappies.

Q3.96 What advice do infected patients require?

The community nurse should advise the patient to follow the general infection control guidance for patients with gastrointestinal infection to prevent spread to family and friends (see Q3.5).

Q3.97 What are the implications for healthcare staff?

If healthcare staff are looking after a patient with *shigella* infection they should follow general infection control guidelines and take basic infection control precautions when handling faeces.

If the healthcare worker has the infection he or she must remain off work until he or she has been symptom free for 48 hours (Working Party of the PHLS *Salmonella* Committee, 1995).

Case history 7

A mother of 3- and 5-year-old girls calls the nurse on Wednesday afternoon for some advice. Her older daughter has been diagnosed as having Shigella sonnei *infection. She has been unwell for a number of days now and is beginning to feel better. The rest of the family has not had any symptoms although the 3-year-old has complained of headaches and tummy ache.*

It is her 3-year-old daughter's birthday party on Saturday and she wonders whether she can still go ahead with it. There will be 20 children coming and 10 adults. The food is to be prepared by herself and her friend and it will be held at the village hall, which has further functions booked for that weekend.

Action

A similar scenario did occur at the beginning of a large outbreak of shigella in a village setting in 1999 (Parry et al., 2001).

The nurse should always seek advice from the CCDC/infection control nurse in public health if this sort of question is asked. There are implications for the other children and adults attending the party and the community at large. The general rule is that anyone with symptoms of diarrhoea and/or vomiting should avoid socializing in large groups until they have been symptom free for 24 to 48 hours.

There is a risk of the infection spreading at the party, particularly as the 3-year-old may well be experiencing the initial symptoms of infection. To protect everyone it is probably best to postpone the party until all are fit and well again.

Summary

Gastrointestinal infections cause considerable morbidity. Prevention of infection through good food and personal hygiene is paramount for everyone, whether travelling or at home.

Chapter 4
Parasitic infections

Introduction

Parasites are organisms that live and thrive on other living beings. Lice are tiny creatures that live on the head and body of human beings. They do not cause significant medical problems but attract inappropriate attention due mostly to society's reaction. Scabies is becoming an important public health problem, especially in institutions such as nursing and residential homes where vulnerable people live together. Threadworms are common amongst children and spread to families, but simple effective remedies are available. Preventive measures can reduce the burden of disease.

Head lice

Q4.1 What are head lice?

Head lice are small (about 1–2 mm long) wingless insects that live on the scalp and feed by sucking blood. They are fully mature after 10 days and can live up to four weeks; in this time the female can lay up to 10 eggs a day. The head louse lays its eggs singly, glued to the hair shaft where the warmth of the scalp will incubate them. The egg is 'tear' shaped and 1 mm in length. The eggs are pink or white and enclosed in a tiny sac, which is firmly attached to the base of the hair shaft, near the scalp (Aston et al., 1998).

The new louse emerges from the egg leaving the empty case (nit) attached to the hair shaft (Aston et al., 1998). Lice become coloured as soon as they feed, and are well camouflaged, reflecting the colour of their surroundings. The empty eggshell (the nit) turns white and becomes more obvious as the growing hair carries it away from the scalp. Nits are the shell of the egg and grow out with the hair unless physically removed by combing. The head louse, pediculus capitis, feeds exclusively by sucking blood from the head. It is host specific and a parasite, spending its entire life on the human head.

Q4.2 How common are head lice?

Infestation with head lice occurs throughout the world. The true prevalence of infection is unknown, although it is probably much lower than the public perception. Although a large number of lice can sometimes be found on a single head, the majority of cases consist of 10 lice or fewer (Muncuoglu et al., 1990; Chosidow et al., 1994).

Q4.3 How is head lice infestation transmitted?

Transmission occurs through close head-to-head contact where the louse walks from one head to another using its powerful claws to hang on to the strand of hair. Head lice like to stay close to the scalp for warmth. They are wingless, cannot fly and they do not jump (see Q4.4).

Q4.4 Who is susceptible?

Head lice do not like the cold surface of skin or clothing and will not live on any other animal but humans. Transmission can occur from person to person within a family, or between children who play together. The whole community is at risk of having head lice. However, most cases are reported in children between the ages of 4 and 11 years (Lindsay, 1993; Vermaak, 1996).

Q4.5 What are the signs and symptoms?

Often there may be no symptoms, so affected people may be unaware they have head lice. However, if left untreated the head may become itchy due to sensitization from the feeding louse, and there is a possibility of secondary infection. Other signs to look for are unusually dirty collars or pillows from louse droppings. Nits and lice can also be seen with the naked eye.

Q4.6 Can you get head lice more than once?

Yes, reinfection does occur.

Q4.7 How are head lice diagnosed?

A diagnosis of head louse infection cannot be made with certainty (no matter how many nits are present, how many reported cases there are in the local community, how bad the itch is reported to be) unless a living, moving louse is found (Aston et al., 1998). The only reliable method of diagnosing current, active infection with head lice is by detection combing (see Q4.8).

Q4.8 What is detection combing?

Detection combing is a process of systematic combing of hair to detect live lice. The community nurse should inform the parent/family member how to detect head lice effectively (Box 4.1), offering support and advice where needed.

Box 4.1 Detection combing

1. Wash the hair well, and then dry with a towel. The hair should be damp, not dripping
2. Make sure there is good light. Daylight is best
3. Comb the hair with an ordinary comb
4. Start with the teeth of the *detection comb* touching the skin of the scalp at the top of the head
5. Draw the comb carefully towards the edge of the hair
6. Look carefully at the teeth of the comb in a good light
7. Do this over and over again from the top of the head to the end of the hair in all directions, working round the head
8. Do this for several minutes. It takes 10 to 15 minutes to do it properly for each head
9. If there are head lice, you will find one or more lice on the teeth of the comb
10. Head lice are little insects with moving legs. They are often not much bigger than a pinhead, but may be as big as a sesame seed
11. Clean the comb under the tap

A plastic detection comb can be purchased from most pharmacies. If the patient finds something and is unsure what it is, you should advise them to stick it on a piece of paper with clear sticky tape to show the practice nurse, school nurse, pharmacist or general practitioner.

Q4.9 What treatments are available to manage head lice?

There are three main groups of insecticidal treatments (pyrethoids, malathion and carbaryl) that are effective against head lice (Burgess, 1996; Vermaak, 1996). Although some degree of resistance to each group has been reported (Burgess, 1990, 1995a, 1995b; Vander et al., 1995), it is less so for carbaryl (Burgess et al., 1992). Unless demonstrated scientifically, resistance is more likely to be due to ovicidal failure, misdiagnosis or faulty treatments. As none of the insecticidal lotions is effective against ova it is recommended that treatment is repeated after seven days.

Insecticidal shampoos are ineffective and should not be used. The three groups of chemicals currently used have a good safety record over many years. The number of reported side-effects recorded by the Adverse Drugs Reactions section of the Committee on Safety of Medicines is small.

Preparations with an alcohol base are contraindicated for people with scalp dermatitis or asthma, who should use aqueous (water) based products. Care must, however, be taken to ensure that they are used in well-ventilated spaces, preferably in the open air, well away from sources of flame and heat such as fires, stoves, cigarettes and hairdryers. Advice should be given to the patient about the care that should be taken to prevent lotion from running over the face and into the eyes. At present carbaryl is available only on prescription whereas the other two products can be purchased over the counter.

Q4.10 How should insecticidal lotion be applied?

Guidelines for the application of lotion are given in Box 4.2.

Box 4.2. Guidelines for the application of lotion

- Lotion should be applied to dry hair
- Part the hair near the top of the head, put a few drops on to the scalp and rub it in. Then part the hair a bit further down the scalp and do the same again
- Do this over and over again until the whole scalp is wet. If the person has long hair lotion does not need to be applied any further than where a ponytail band would be tied
- Use enough lotion — at least one small bottle for each head, more if the hair is thick. Use all the lotion
- Keep the lotion out of eyes and off the face. One way is to hold a cloth over the face
- Let the lotion dry on the hair
- Some lotions are flammable, so keep well away from flames, cigarettes, stoves and other sources of heat
- Do not use a hairdryer
- Leave on hair for the recommended time
- Comb through the hair using a fine-toothed comb or a 'nit comb'
- Wash lotion off hair using ordinary shampoo
- After treatment continue to wet-comb throughout the week to check for head lice or eggs
- Treat again seven days later in the same way with the same lotion
- Wet comb a day or two after the second treatment to check treatment has been successful
- If there are still living, moving lice, treatment has failed and an alternative treatment should be used

---

Q4.11 Are there any alternative methods of treatment?

A mechanical removal of lice by wet combing the hair after using conditioner – popularly known as 'Bug Busting' – has been employed in treating head lice and controlling spread. This technique involves applying a handful of conditioner to wet hair and then using a plastic comb to comb the hair in a manner similar to detection combing. A treatment session takes 20–30 minutes and has to be repeated every three or four days for a minimum of two weeks. Its effectiveness has to date not been substantiated by any authoritative scientific work. There are anecdotal reports of both its success and failure. However, when insecticidal treatment fails it would be reasonable to try this method.

Q4.12 Do repellents work for head lice?

Proprietary products that claim to repel lice should not be recommended. Even if they were effective in protecting the individual from infection, they do not deal with the control of lice in the population, and do not treat existing infections.

Q4.13 How can head lice infestation be prevented ?

Regular grooming will help in prevention. Frequent and vigorous combing will damage lice and disturb their environment. Identifying the early signs of infestation by regularly checking the family's hair will help to prevent lice becoming a problem (see Box 4.1). Using a detector comb on damp hair ensures early detection of live lice (Burgess et al., 1992).

Q4.14 Is tea tree oil helpful in preventing reinfestation?

There is no evidence that tea tree oil is useful in getting rid of head lice.

Q4.15 Does the school have a responsibility to ensure all children are treated for head lice?

The responsibility for treatment rests with the parents.

Q4.16 Should children with long hair be advised to tie it in a plait?

There is no evidence that this helps in reducing transmission between children.

Q4.17 Can head lice be transmitted via headwear?

Head lice are not usually transmitted via headwear.

Case history 8

Helen Brown has come home from school with a note saying that there has been an outbreak of head lice in her class. The note advises parents to check their children's hair and treat anyone who has lice. Mrs Brown visits the practice nurse that day and insists that her whole family is given a prescription immediately for head lice.

Action

The practice nurse reassures Mrs Brown that the infection rarely leads to any harm and there is no need to panic. The practice nurse then explains what head lice are, and the different methods of control and treatment. Mrs Brown explains that she is a busy working mother and would like to be prescribed lotion that gets rid of the lice with minimum effort from her. The practice nurse explains that there are products available both to buy over the counter and to obtain on prescription and advises Mrs Brown about the different treatments. She then explains that head lice treatment should be given only to those people who have actually got live lice on their heads. Mrs Brown was not aware of this and thought that the whole family should be treated.

The practice nurse then explains how to check for head lice, and to prevent and control further outbreaks. Mrs Brown collects a leaflet from reception about detection combing. The leaflet clearly states that if she is unable to see lice then she should not treat. The practice nurse provides the family with a leaflet and the contact number for the community infection control nurse or school nurse for further information and advice.

Scabies

Q4.18 What is scabies?

Scabies is an itchy, infectious condition of the skin caused by infestation by mites.

Q4.19 How is it caused?

The cause of scabies is a mite called *Sarcoptes scabiei*. It is a small eight-legged disc-shaped parasite that lives in burrows in the outer layer of the skin. The mites cannot be seen by the naked eye.

Q4.20 How common is it?

Scabies is common throughout the world and an estimated 300 million cases occur each year. The true prevalence of the disease in the UK is unknown as it is not a notifiable disease. Anecdotal evidence would suggest that sporadic cases are common in both sexes and in all ages. There has certainly been an increase in reports of outbreaks in schools, long-stay wards in hospitals, residential homes and units caring for patients with AIDS (Barrett and Morse, 1993; Figueroa, 1998). Scabies is also shown to have a cyclical rise in incidence roughly every 20 years (Downs et al., 1999).

Q4.21 What are the symptoms?

Classical scabies

The main symptom of scabies is itching, particularly at night. The itch of scabies is related to an allergic response to the mite or its products. Classical scabies infection is found in healthy people with normal immune systems and usually involves few mites. Burrows on the skin, which are raised, skin-coloured or grey and usually only a few millimetres in length are a classical sign. They are most common in finger webs, or on the sides of the fingers, flexor surfaces of the wrists and elbows, male genitalia or women's breasts (Chosidow, 2000). In healthy adults the face and skull are rarely involved. In infants, burrows are common on the palms and may occur on the face and skull (Figueroa, 1998). Because of the intense itching secondary bacterial infection is common, especially on the hands, and may be a presenting feature.

Norwegian scabies

The symptoms of scabies in those with an impaired immune system (HIV/AIDS, systemic steroid therapy, organ transplant recipients) are quite different and usually involve a large number of mites. They may have crusted (Norwegian) scabies, which is characterized by hyperkeratotic legions, usually on the hands, scalp, feet and ears. The nails are often involved and may be disfigured. The rash may not itch. Patients with Norwegian scabies are extremely infectious and can be the cause of outbreaks of classical scabies amongst close contacts.

Q4.22 What is the incubation period?

From exposure to development of symptoms can take between three and six weeks. However, because it is an allergic response and the patient may already be sensitized, symptoms may develop after only a few days following reinfection.

Q4.23 How is it transmitted and what is the infectious period?

Scabies is transmitted by direct skin-to-skin contact. Sexual transmission is also common, as is non-sexual spread amongst family groups (Chosidow, 2000). In classical scabies the average number of female mites is around 12. As long as mites are present the person is infectious. Crusted scabies is highly infectious as there may be many thousand mites. The more parasites on an individual the greater the likelihood of transmission.

Q4.24 How is scabies diagnosed?

Apart from clinical signs and symptoms, definitive diagnosis is made by microscopic examination of mites, eggs or mite faeces by taking skin scrapings. Often it is not possible to get a firm diagnosis and a history of nocturnal itching, together with symptomatic family members or partners, should suggest the disease.

Q4.25 What is the natural history of scabies?

Infections with scabies require treatment. The available treatment is effective and there are no long-term sequelae. However, successful treatment does not give long-term protection and reinfection is common. If untreated, scratching leads to secondary bacterial infection.

Q4.26 How is scabies treated?

Scabicidal treatment is available (Effectiveness Matters, 1999) and is effective, which renders an individual symptom free and non-infectious. There are a number of scabicidal treatments but those used commonly in the United Kingdom include malathion 0.5% and permethrin 5% dermal cream. Both are available in aqueous or alcohol preparations. Aqueous treatment is recommended as alcohol may cause irritation. Because of the long incubation period all close contacts and members of the household of the index case should be treated simultaneously. Resistance is uncommon and both malathion and permethrin treatments are clinically effective (PHLS 2000b). Most treatment failures can be attributed to inadequate application (Effectiveness Matters, 1999). Treatment should be applied to the whole body, paying particular attention to the webs of the fingers and toes and brushing lotion on the end of the nails. In the case of infants and young children up to two years old, the elderly, the immuno-compromised and those who have experienced treatment failure, applications should be extended to the scalp, neck, face and ears. It is recommended that treatment should be applied twice, one week apart (BNF, 2001). It is important to emphasize that hands should not be washed, and if they are the treatment should be reapplied. The manufacturer's instructions should be followed as to how long to leave the lotion on for (eight to 12 hours for permethrin and 24 hours for malathion).

Patients with crusted (Norwegian) scabies may require two or three applications before they are rid of mites. Ivermectin in a dose of 200 micrograms per kg body weight as a single dose is a useful treatment for crusted scabies (Offidani et al., 1999). It is not yet licensed for use in the treatment of scabies in the UK but may be obtained on a named patient basis from the manufacturer. Ivermectin may also be useful in nursing homes where outbreaks can be difficult to control. However, a recent report on the use of the drug in controlling an outbreak of scabies in a residential unit for the elderly suggested a possibility of excess deaths amongst the residents (Barwell and Shields, 1997). Other published reports have challenged this conclusion and have documented the use of ivermectin in elderly individuals without any adverse effects (Coyne and Addiss, 1997; del Guidice and Marty, 1999).

Although manufacturers do not recommend treatment during pregnancy there is no definite evidence that any of the currently employed topical scabicides has been harmful during pregnancy following appropriate use (PHLS, 2000b). Itching may persist for two to three weeks after treatment even if treatment has been successful. However, persistence of itching for a longer period needs investigation as it may be due to treatment failure.

Q4.27 What about bedding and clothing?

Scabies is spread from person to person by direct physical contact. There is very little chance of transfer from clothing and bedding as mites found in the environment die quickly and do not present a risk (Effectiveness Matters, 1999). Washing bed linen and clothes in a hot wash is adequate to get rid of the mite.

Q4.28 How can scabies be prevented?

Scabies can be prevented by limiting contact with the mite. This entails early diagnosis, adequate contact tracing and treatment of all those who have prolonged skin-to-skin contact with the infected person. Advice can be sought from the local communicable disease team.

Case history 9

A staff nurse from a local nursing home is concerned that in the last week or so four residents have developed an itchy rash and a staff member has been sent off duty with the same symptoms. The nurse suspects that it might be an infectious rash and asks for advice.

Action

It is not uncommon for the elderly to have a rash. First, arrangements should be made for the local general practitioner to see the patients and staff and confirm the diagnosis of scabies. If there are any doubts, it would be prudent to get the help of a dermatologist. If scabies is confirmed the patients, relatives and staff should be reassured that it is a treatable disease and provided with information in the form of leaflets. All close contacts, i.e. family or friends of all the residents and staff, should be identified. How many staff and residents are treated will depend on the closeness of the contact. If it is a nursing home with two separate buildings and staff and residents do not mix with each other then it is possible to treat just those affected. In other situations the whole nursing home population including staff would need to be treated.

Adequate lotion for everyone must be ordered and a date set for everyone to treat themselves. Those who are less able to do so should be offered help. All identified contacts should be treated on the same day.

There is no need to have a hot bath before starting treatment. The prescribed treatment (permethrin or malathion) should be applied from the jaw line downwards, including behind the ears and at the top of the neck (see Q 4.26). It is necessary to ensure that the finger webs and all body creases are carefully treated. The fingernails should be cut short, scrubbed clean then the lotion or cream brushed under the nails. If hands are washed, the treatment should be reapplied to the washed areas. Preparation should be left on for the recommended period and when treatment is completed the lotion can be washed off in a shower or bath. After this the nursing home needs to monitor very carefully all the residents and staff to make sure that there has been no treatment failure. Some patients with scabies may continue itching for a couple of weeks after treatment, and soothing creams can be applied to alleviate these symptoms.

Threadworms (*Enterobius vermiculari*)

Q4.29 What are threadworms?

Threadworms (also known as pin worms) are small, whitish, threadlike worms (nematodes) which are 5–12mm long (Donaldson and Donaldson, 2000). They live in the caecum, small and large intestine of humans.

Q4.30 How common are they?

Threadworm infection is not a notifiable disease but is known to occur worldwide (Chin, 2000). It is estimated that up to 15 million people in the UK are infected, most of whom are children (Donaldson and Donaldson, 2000).

Q4.31 What is the incubation period?

The incubation period is long, two to six weeks, because of the time it takes for the worm to complete its life cycle (Figure 4.1). In addition, worms may inhabit the gut for a period of time without the host developing symptoms.

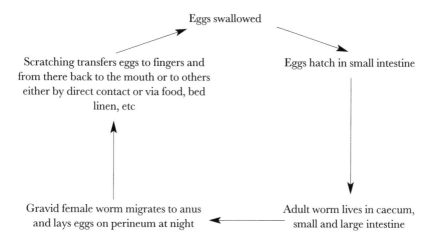

Source: Donaldson and Donaldson (2000).

Figure 4.1 Life cycle of threadworms.

Q4.32 How are they transmitted?

The adult female lays her eggs around the anal area at night. This causes intense itching. When the area is scratched eggs can be transferred to fingers. The eggs can then be transferred either directly to the mouth (Sinclair, 1997), or indirectly to another person. The eggs are capable of survival for a number of days on fomites and in dust if the environment is moist and cool (Donaldson and Donaldson, 2000). However, person-to-person transmission is most common.

Q4.33 Who is susceptible?

Anyone is susceptible, but children are most likely to be infected. They are also more likely to put their fingers in their mouths after contact with objects or toys touched by other children. Close contacts of a case, such as household contacts, have an increased risk of becoming infected themselves compared with casual acquaintances (Chin, 2000).

Q4.34 What are the signs and symptoms?

The most common symptoms include intense perianal itching, leading to disturbed sleep (see Q4.32). Often there may be no symptoms but adult worms may be seen on the stools as tiny white threads. The infection may rarely lead to vulvovaginitis, salpingitis and pelvic and liver granulomata (Chin, 2000).

Q4.35 What is the natural history?

The worm's life cycle is about six weeks. In order for the symptoms to continue after this period, there has to be reinfection of the host, i.e. further eggs being transferred from anus to mouth. An individual worm lives for about two months.

Q4.36 Can you get infected with threadworms again?

Yes. Previous infection does not produce immunity against further infection.

Q4.37 How is the infection diagnosed?

Infection with threadworms is diagnosed through clinical history. The most reliable method of confirming diagnosis is through identification under a microscope of eggs retrieved using transparent sticky tape around the anus (threadworm egg collection kits may be available from the microbiology laboratory).

Q4.38 How is it treated?

Anti-worm medicines (anthelmintics) can be prescribed by the GP or can be bought from the chemist. Treatment will be successful if the infected person and his or her close household contacts are all treated simultaneously (Sinclair, 1997) and strict hygiene precautions are observed.

Mebendazole 100 mg as a single dose is the treatment of choice for adults and children over 2 years of age. If reinfection takes place a second dose two to three weeks after the initial treatment is recommended (BNF, 2001). Mebendazole is not licensed for use in children under 2 years of age.

The alternative is to prescribe piperazine powder in infants aged over 3 months. The whole family should be treated even if they are not experiencing any symptoms. Although treatment is effective, hygiene measures must also be taken to prevent reinfection and ensure eradication of the worms and eggs. Following treatment, all bedding should be changed and rooms cleaned thoroughly to remove dust. Young children who have symptoms should wear underwear or pyjamas in bed to prevent them from scratching their naked bottoms during the night and recontaminating their hands (National Prescribing Centre 1999).

Q4.39 How is it prevented?

Threadworm infection is prevented by scrupulous hygiene. This includes the following:

1. Everyone should remember to wash his or her hands after using the lavatory and before eating.
2. The nails should be kept short.
3. The infected individuals should stop putting his or her hands in the mouth.
4. Bed linen should be changed regularly.
5. Clean nightwear should be worn every day.
6. A morning bath or shower should be taken to remove newly laid eggs.
7. Everyone in the household should keep up these precautions for six weeks.

Case history 10

A local primary school has had a number of parents reporting that their children have got threadworms. The head teacher asks the school nurse for some advice.

Action

The school nurse can reassure the head teacher that this is a common, non-life-threatening infection. The school does not need to close. However, parents might appreciate an information leaflet about threadworms. In addition children should have access to running water, soap and paper towels and hand washing should be supervised, particularly before lunch and after using the lavatory. Infected children can return to school when they have been treated.

Summary

Although parasitic infections cause social stigma and concern, they are not life threatening. All community nurses have an important role in reassuring the public, and providing information leaflets and support.

Chapter 5
Respiratory infections

Introduction

Respiratory infections are a common cause of morbidity and mortality, especially amongst the elderly. Influenza is responsible for many deaths every winter. For those at high risk, a vaccine is available to prevent infection. New drugs are becoming available which may reduce the severity of illness. Tuberculosis is a worldwide disease and, after a relatively stable situation, case numbers have been increasing in the United Kingdom. Although effective therapy is available, some bacteria are developing resistance to routinely used anti-tubercular drugs.

Influenza

Q5.1 What is influenza?

The influenza virus causes an acute viral infection of the respiratory tract. There are three types of influenza virus: types A and B which cause epidemics, and type C which is less common and is associated with sporadic cases. Outbreaks of influenza A virus occur in most years and are the usual cause of epidemics. Influenza B can also cause outbreaks but these tend to be less frequent. Influenza viruses are labile due to changes that occur from season to season through a process known as antigenic shift. This leads to the emergence of a new subtype to which the population has little immunity (see Q5.7).

Q5.2 How common is it?

Influenza derives its importance from the rapidity with which epidemics evolve (DoH, 1997). During the past 100 years or so there have been pandemics in 1889, 1918, 1957 and 1968. Clinical attack rates during epidemics range from 10 to 20 per cent in the general community to more than 50 per cent in closed populations, for example nursing homes (Chin, 2000) (see Q5.6). Epidemics usually happen in the winter months in temperate climates, and in the rainy season in tropical climates. However, there have been sporadic cases and outbreaks reported in any month of the year.

Epidemics are generally associated with excess deaths mainly among the elderly (Ashley et al., 1996). Even in winters when incidence is low, 3000–4000 deaths may be attributed to influenza infections in the UK (DoH, 2000) (see Q5.7).

Q5.3 What is the incubation period?

The incubation period is short, usually between one and four days.

Q5.4 What are the symptoms of influenza?

The infection is characterized by:

- the abrupt onset of fever;
- chills;
- headache;
- myalgia;
- sometimes prostration;
- a dry cough;
- there may be a sore throat.

It is usually a self-limiting disease with recovery in two to seven days, but can be a serious illness and may be complicated by bronchitis, secondary bacterial pneumonia and otitis media in children (Chin, 2000).

Q5.5 How infectious is influenza?

Influenza is highly infectious during the period of illness. Adults are infectious for the first three to five days after clinical onset, and children a little longer, until about seven days (Chin, 2000).

Q5.6 How is it transmitted?

The influenza virus is transmitted by airborne spread and directly by objects contaminated with secretions from the nose. Humans are the primary reservoir for human infections. The infection spreads rapidly in confined spaces, and among crowded populations. Transmission may also occur by indirect contact as the influenza virus may persist for hours, particularly when it is cold and in the presence of low humidity.

Q5.7 Who is susceptible to influenza?

When a new subtype of influenza appears, all children and adults are at risk. Infection produces immunity to the specific infecting virus. It can spread rapidly, especially in institutions such as nursing and residential homes. People of all ages are at risk of influenza, although the most vulnerable are the elderly and those who have chronic diseases, including asthma; chronic heart disease; chronic renal failure; diabetes mellitus; and immunosuppression due to disease or treatment (DoH, 1997; Fleming et al., 1997).

Q5.8 How is influenza treated?

Treatment is mainly to relieve the symptoms, i.e. antipyretics, pain killing drugs and antihistamines. Amantidine hypochloride is an effective antiviral agent against influenza A and has been used prophylactically to control outbreaks. Zanamivir is available to treat influenza A and B. If given within 48 hours after onset of symptoms it can reduce the duration of symptoms.

Q5.9 How is influenza prevented?

There is little value in isolation because of the large number of cases that occur in epidemics. Education is extremely important in an outbreak of influenza, ensuring that people are aware of signs and symptoms. This includes encouraging people with influenza to self-medicate and stay at home to prevent spread of the virus (see Q5.4–Q5.6, Q5.13).

Q5.10 Is there a vaccine available?

In recent years the most significant method of prevention and control of influenza has been the introduction of the influenza vaccine (DoH, 1996a). Influenza immunization is recommended for the groups listed in Box 5.1.

Published studies have found that only 40 per cent of these high-risk individuals received vaccination annually (Nguyen-Van-Tam and Nicholson, 1993). There is published evidence that influenza vaccine is effective in reducing mortality in older people in the community and individuals

---

Box 5.1 Patients recommended to have active immunization

---

1. Those of all ages with:
    * chronic heart disease
    * chronic respiratory disease, including asthma
    * chronic renal disease
    * diabetes mellitus
    * immunosuppression due to disease or treatment
2. All aged 65 years and over
3. Those living in long-stay residential and nursing homes or other long-stay facilities

Source: DoH (1996a).

---

who are at high risk (Ahmed et al., 1995; Fleming et al., 1995). General practitioners are encouraged to vaccinate all patients aged 65 and over, to reduce the morbidity of the disease (NHS Centre for Reviews and Dissemination, 1996).

Influenza immunization offers a 70–80 per cent protection against infection in healthy young adults, though in the elderly it may be less effective (DoH, 1996a). The vaccine should be given each year before the influenza season. Immunization should be considered for those working with the elderly, the immunocompromised or the very young, and health-care workers (DoH, 2000).

The influenza vaccine is an inactive vaccine in a dose of 0.5 ml (in adults) given by intramuscular or deep subcutaneous injection into the deltoid muscle. Children below 12 years of age receive two injections (0.5 ml for 4- to 12-year-olds and 0.25 ml for those aged 6 months to 3 years) four to six weeks apart when receiving influenza vaccine for the first time.

The vaccine is usually well tolerated. Localized soreness does occur around the injection site. There have been reports of fever and malaise, usually beginning about six to 12 hours after the injection. Vaccination is contraindicated in people with anaphylactic hypersensitivity to hens' eggs.

Q5.11 Can the flu jab cause flu?

The flu jab is not a live vaccine therefore cannot cause flu. It is usually well tolerated apart from occasional soreness at the injection site. Very rarely it can cause fever, malaise, myalgia and/or arthralgia lasting up to 48 hours.

Because the vaccine is developed to protect against a specific strain(s) of virus, there is always the possibility that a person will contract a different influenza virus.

Q5.12 What is the difference between flu and a cold?

During a cold a sore throat, stuffy nose and sneezing are common, with mild aches and pains and chest discomfort – a raised temperature is rare. Occasionally complications occur such as sinus congestion or earache. The illness is mild and short lasting.

In flu there is characteristically a high temperature lasting three to four days, headache is prominent, there are general aches and pains, and fatigue and weakness are severe. Exhaustion is early and prominent and chest discomfort is common, which can lead to bronchitis or pneumonia and in some cases, especially in the elderly, can be life threatening (see Q5.4)

Q5.13 Is it safe to go to school or work with flu symptoms?

Patients with flu should be advised to rest at home when they have symptoms.

Q5.14 Are special infection control procedures needed when running a flu jab clinic?

There is no need for any special infection control procedures. Universal precautions should be adhered to (see Q1.14)

Case history 11

A practice nurse is contacted by a 28-year-old women with a request for flu vaccination. She has visited the general practitioner who has stated that the patient does not need to have the flu vaccine.

Action

The practice nurse requests further information from the woman. She ascertains that the woman is young, fit and healthy with no underlying illness. She is not employed working with people; she is a housewife with no children. The practice nurse explains that she is at low risk and that the flu vaccine is recommended for people over the age of 65 years, those people at 'high risk', people in institutional care and people who are immunocompromised. The woman is reassured that she does not fall into the risk category for serious disease, and is given advice about self-care if she does contract flu.

Tuberculosis (TB)

Q5.15 What is TB?

TB is a chronic infection that can involve many parts of the body. The most common site of infection is the lungs (pulmonary tuberculosis) but it can also cause infection in the lymph nodes, pleura, pericardium, kidneys, bones, meninges (causing meningitis), joints, larynx, skin, intestines, peritoneum and eyes. Infection not invading the lungs is known as extrapulmonary tuberculosis (Chin, 2000).

Q5.16 What causes the disease?

TB is caused by Mycobacterium bacteria. The three main Mycobacterium types are *mycobacterium tuberculosis, mycobacterium bovis* and *mycobacterium africanum*. In humans it is not possible to distinguish between the different Mycobacterium strains clinically, radiologically or pathologically. The causative organism can be differentiated only by its microbiological characteristics (Hardie and Watson, 1992).

   The main reservoir for pathogenic Mycobacterium is primarily humans, rarely primates (Chin, 2000) and in some areas diseased cattle, badgers, swine and other mammals (Hardie and Watson, 1992).

Q5.17 How common is TB?

In England and Wales the number of cases of TB has been declining for some decades (Figure 5.1) (see Q5.31). In the 1990s around 6000 cases of TB were notified annually, with a slight increase in the past few years. Pulmonary TB continues to be the most common site affected and is twice as common as non-respiratory infection (Figure 5.2).

Q5.18 How is TB transmitted?

Most commonly it is passed from people with pulmonary or laryngeal TB via the airborne route (i.e. coughing) to susceptible people who are in prolonged close contact with the infected person (see Q5.20).

   Extrapulmonary TB is not infectious except where there are exudating lesions (see Q5.23). *Mycobacterium bovis* (bovine TB) may be passed from infected cattle either via airborne spread if the animal has lung lesions or through drinking infected unpasteurized milk (Mims et al., 1995).

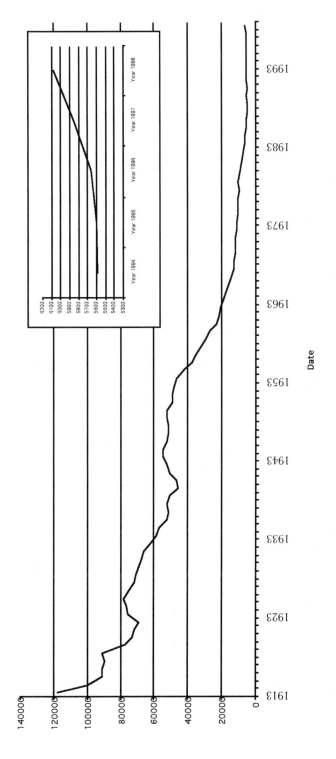

Figure 5.1 Tuberculosis: respiratory and non-respiratory notification England and Wales 1993–98.
Source: Public Health Laboratory Service Communicable Disease Surveillance Centre (2001).

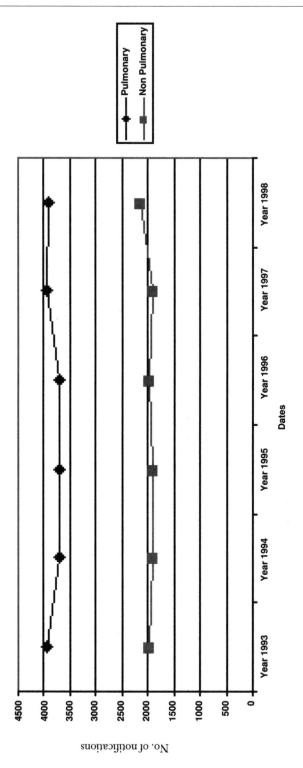

Figure 5.2 Tuberculosis: pulmonary and non-pulmonary notifications, England and Wales 1993–98. *Source:* Public Health Laboratory Service Communicable Disease Surveillance Centre (2001).

Q5.19 How infectious is it?

Patients who are sputum positive, i.e. have tubercle bacilli in their sputum, are infectious to others (see Q5.32). However, these individuals usually become non-infectious after two weeks of standard treatment including rifampicin and isoniazid (Joint Committee of the British Thoracic Society, 2000) (see Q5.24, Q5.25).

Patients who have been diagnosed as having TB involving other parts of their body, i.e. extrapulmonary, are not regarded as infectious to others (Wilson, 1995).

Q5.20 Who is susceptible?

Anyone who has prolonged and close contact with an infectious person or animal and has no prior immunity to the organism is susceptible to TB (Chin, 2000). Those with inadequate immune systems, people with HIV and the homeless are at increased risk of acquiring TB infection.

Q5.21 What is the incubation period?

Incubation is four to 12 weeks, although the initial infection may go unnoticed. A localized reaction in the lung occurs, which is about the size of a small coin. This is called the Ghon focus. From here the organisms are carried to neighbouring lymph glands, which become enlarged. This is known as the primary complex and usually heals spontaneously.

In most infections the disease process stops at this stage. The immune system and body defences seal off the complex by depositing calcium salts which, over time, harden off and imprison the bacilli. These can be seen on X-ray as dense small shadows and indicate past infection that has been overcome – they are not a cause for concern (see Q5.23).

If the body's defences are not successful, the lesions will continue to develop and become soft, known as caseous (cheesy) degeneration. Bacteria can escape from these tubercles in large numbers and spread to any part of the body (Meers et al., 1995).

Q5.22 What are the symptoms?

Pulmonary TB

The most common symptom is a cough, initially quite mild but getting progressively worse, which does not respond to the usually prescribed broad-spectrum antibiotics. There may be blood in the sputum as a result of erosion of the lung and neighbouring blood vessels. Patients may also experience fever, weight loss and night sweats, which may be attributable to the impact of disease on the body (Chin, 2000).

Extrapulmonary TB

Symptoms of extrapulmonary TB will vary depending on the organ involved: this may be the meninges, lymph nodes, bones and joints, kidney and urinary tract, gastrointestinal and skin.

Q5.23 How is TB diagnosed?

Apart from the clinical history and signs and symptoms on examination (see Q5.22), chest X-ray, tuberculin testing and bacteriological examination of sputum help to diagnose TB.

Chest X-ray

The X-ray of the chest may show signs of infection in the lungs, a cavity or collapsed lung, or miliary TB (fine mottling, symmetrically distributed throughout both lung fields).

Tuberculin testing (Heaf or Mantoux)

This is a skin test that assesses an individual's sensitivity to tuberculin protein (see Q5.27).

Sputum or bronchial washings

These may isolate acid-fast bacilli. Sputum also has to be sent for culture of mycobacterium tuberculosis (see Q5.25).

Q5.24 How is TB treated?

TB is treated in two phases. The aim of phase one is to decrease the number of bacteria as quickly as possible to stop the emergence of resistant strains.

The drugs of choice (assuming that the patient does not have a resistant form of TB) comprise the daily use of isoniazid, rifampicin and pyrazinamide. This phase usually lasts two months. The second phase, which lasts about four months, involves the use of rifampicin and isoniazid (BNF, 2001) (see Q5.30).

Patients being treated with rifampicin should be informed that urine, faeces, saliva, sputum, sweat and tears may be coloured orange (Guy's Hospital, 1994).

Q5.25 How is the spread of TB controlled?

Surveillance

TB is a notifiable disease and all cases must be reported to the local public health department by the diagnosing doctor. All parts of the NHS are required to maintain and improve the health of the population, including arrangements for the control of communicable disease (HSG, 1993). Even so, it is recognized that there is under-reporting of TB (Brown et al., 1995).

Contact tracing

Close contacts of a case of TB are followed up by the local chest clinic (see Q5.26). This may involve a tuberculin test (Heaf/Mantoux) (see Q5.27) and a chest X-ray (see Q5.23).

Treatment

Those identified as having TB are commenced on treatment and followed up to ensure treatment is effective and successful (see Q5.24, Q5.30). In some cases the infected individual may be hospitalized and isolated until no longer infectious, to protect the population. Patients with sputum-positive TB who have undergone two weeks of therapy with standard anti-tuberculous drugs are not infectious even if mycobacterium can be seen in their sputum.

Microbiological typing

All mycobacterial isolates are sent for typing to a central laboratory so that the organism can be monitored. This is particularly useful in situations where it is thought that an outbreak has occurred and for the identification of resistant strains.

Q5.26 Who are close contacts?

Close contacts are people who have prolonged, intimate contact with the index case, e.g. family, kissing contacts.

Q5.27 What is a Heaf/Mantoux test?

A Heaf or Mantoux test assesses the individual's sensitivity to tuber-culin protein; the greater the strength of the tuberculin reaction the more likely an individual is to have active disease (see Q5.29). For those with no reaction, BCG immunization is recommended to protect against TB.

Q5.28 Is there a vaccine to prevent TB?

Yes, BCG (Bacillus Calmette-Guerin) is a live vaccine that has been shown to have efficacy of 70–80 per cent in protecting against tubercu-losis when given to British children. In the UK BCG is recommended at birth for those at high risk (those with a history of somebody in the family with TB, or from countries with a high prevalence of TB, e.g. the Indian subcontinent). BCG is also routinely given to children (aged 10–14 years) who have no reaction to a Heaf test as part of the school BCG programme. In addition, BCG is also recommended for those at high risk, including:

- health service staff;
- veterinary staff;
- staff working in residential settings;
- close contacts of known TB cases;
- immigrants from countries with a high prevalence of TB;
- long-stay visitors to countries with a high prevalence of TB (DoH, 1996a).

Q5.29 Who does the Heaf/Mantoux test?

The technique for vaccination and interpretation of the Heaf test requires specialist knowledge. Therefore, Heaf testing and vaccination are performed by specially trained doctors and nurses, usually found in school health teams, chest departments and some occupational health departments. The procedure is not performed in general practice.

In 1999 and 2000 there was a national shortage of BCG and the schools programme was stopped. It recommenced in September 2001 when BCG supplies were readily available again.

Q5.30 Can TB be treated successfully?

Yes, although the treatment, usually three separate antibiotics, has to be taken for at least six months. Ensuring that patients complete the course plays an important part in controlling the disease and preventing resistance in the organism (see Q5.24).

In some countries, patients' compliance with treatment has caused great concern. The main problem is that once the individual begins to feel better he or she stops treatment because of the unpleasant side-effects that may occur. To prevent this from happening the use of directly observed therapy (DOT) is recommended for those at risk of non-adherence with the treatment (Joint Tuberculosis Committee of the British Thoracic Society, 2000). In these cases the patient is handed his or her medication and is observed taking the medication by the healthcare worker.

Q5.31 Is it true that TB is becoming more prevalent?

In England and Wales total annual notifications fell following the introduction of drug treatment and BCG vaccination in the 1950s (see Figure 5.1). However, the most significant decline in cases occurred around the turn of the twentieth century onwards and is attributed to better overall health of the population as a result of improved social conditions such as general sanitation (Wilson, 1995).

Since 1987 the number of notifications of TB has gradually risen. This may be due to a number of reasons, such as increasing numbers of people with HIV who are more susceptible to TB; increasing numbers of immigrants from countries where the prevalence of TB continues to rise; increasing numbers of people living in overcrowded conditions or who are homeless (Hayward and Watson, 1995).

Globally, TB kills two million people a year. In 1993 the World Health Organisation declared TB a global emergency and estimated that, if control is not strengthened, between the years 2000 and 2020 one billion people will be newly infected, 200 million people will get sick and 35 million will die from TB worldwide.

Q5.32 A colleague at work has been diagnosed with TB. Do I need antibiotics?

All cases of TB should be notified through the Public Health Department so that contact tracing can be initiated. If the index case is sputum smear positive, work colleagues may well require follow up (see Q5.19).

Q5.33 There have been reports of outbreaks of TB in schools and colleges where the children have been vaccinated. Doesn't the BCG offer immunity to the disease?

The BCG has an efficacy of 70–80 per cent.

Q5.34 When someone is initially diagnosed, does he or she have to be isolated for two weeks until the treatment is established?

If the index case is sputum smear positive he or she may be nursed in isolation in hospital or advised not to socialize with strangers for two weeks, to allow antibiotic therapy time to work.

Summary

Community staff need to be aware of the increasing incidence of TB, and be able to recognize potential cases. Any person who complains of weight loss, night sweats and a cough should be referred immediately to the GP.

Chapter 6
Other common infections

Introduction

This chapter looks at other important infections, some recent (MRSA), those amongst which vaccines have made some progress (meningitis) but continue to be important health issues, and others (impetigo, shingles) commonly seen by general practitioners.

MRSA

Q6.1 What is methicillin-resistant *Staphylococcus aureus* (MRSA) ?

Staphylococcus aureus is a human commensal present on the skin of approximately 30 per cent of people, and is particularly common among those working in the clinical environment (Siu, 1994). It is a gram-positive organism that is capable of rapid spread and can cause serious infections in vulnerable people, although it will be present on others with no ill effect.

Most strains of this bacterium are sensitive to many antibiotics and infections can be treated effectively. *Staphylococcus aureus* that are resistant to an antibiotic called methicillin are referred to as methicillin-resistant *Staphylococcus aureus* or MRSA. MRSA has been linked to hospital-acquired infections since the early 1960s.

MRSA rarely presents a danger to the general public. It is an opportunistic agent, which infects patients by several modes of transmission and spreads among those who are severely ill, many of whom have received antibiotics previously (Siu, 1994).

MRSA strains were described first in 1961 but may have occurred naturally before the advent of methicillin. Methicillin resistance in staphylococci was reported in 1961 (Duckworth, 1993). Most patients from whom MRSA is isolated are colonized rather than infected with this organism (see Q6.2).

The incidence of MRSA has increased over the past three decades and although outbreaks have been uncommon, sporadic cases have continued to be reported throughout the UK since the late 1980s. MRSA occurs worldwide and can be found in many healthcare environments, with the importation of strains from other countries remaining a problem for healthcare workers within the UK (Sanderson, 1994).

Q 6.2 What is difference between colonization and infection?

Infection with MRSA will lead to illness including swelling, redness and increase in temperature of the affected part, leading to pus formation. *Colonization* with MRSA means the presence of this organism in the nose, back of the throat or skin without any illness (see Q6.7).

Q6.3 How is MRSA transmitted?

Transient carriage of MRSA on staff hands is the main route of spread, and cross-infection in wards is difficult to prevent by routine measures (Working Party, 1998). Outbreaks of infection both in hospital and in the community occur as a result of poor compliance with hand washing. Although MRSA is capable of spreading by airborne transmission or on contaminated equipment (Taylor, 1990) the most common route is by contact between people.

Q6.4 Who is susceptible to MRSA?

MRSA can create major problems for patients in hospital who are severely ill, including patients in intensive care units, special care baby units, maternity units, burns units, operating theatres and surgical wards. In these areas patients are often immunocompromised and have a higher risk of developing infection, which in rare cases can lead to death (Duckworth, 1993). Some nursing homes have also experienced problems with this bacterium.

Risk factors for acquiring MRSA include:

* previous hospitalization;
* intravenous lines;
* pressure sores;
* underlying disease;
* recent antibiotic therapy (Cafferkey et al., 1988).

However, despite the potential to cause serious infection, most MRSA colonize rather than infect the skin and mucous membranes (French et al., 1990) (see Q6.2). In the community the risk of infection from a colonized person to others is minimal as most people are generally healthy. Those who are vulnerable to infection, such as patients in hospital and the elderly, are at higher risk.

Q6.5 What are the signs and symptoms of MRSA?

The colonized patient with MRSA will show no signs or symptoms. However, if a patient has fever and inflammation associated with the presence of MRSA he or she is infected. MRSA is usually discovered when an infected wound fails to respond to common antibiotic therapy.

Q6.6 How is MRSA diagnosed?

The diagnosis of MRSA infection is made by microbiological tests – when the organism is isolated by culture from material taken from the lesion, blood or body fluid. A wound swab can be kept overnight if stored in the correct specimen container (see Q1.17).

Q6.7 How is MRSA treated?

The treatment of patients affected with MRSA falls into two categories:

1. treatment of colonization
2. treatment of infection.

Treatment of colonization

Widespread colonization presents a problem for both hospital and community healthcare staff (see Q6.2–Q6.4).

There is good evidence to suggest that carriage of MRSA by patients and hospital staff provides an important source for subsequent spread. Therefore an attempt should be made to eradicate colonization in hospitalized patients and healthcare staff (Working Party, 1998).

Topical mupirocin 2% applied two or three times a day for five days is effective in eradicating colonization. However, patients who live in low-risk areas, i.e. nursing homes and patients in their own home, can return from hospital as colonized patients without significant risk to the community. At this point universal hygienic precautions are required (Duckworth and Heathcock, 1995) (see Q1.14).

Treatment of infection

Topical antibiotic treatment (mupirocin 2%) for MRSA is the recommended treatment for patients with infected wounds and skin lesions. In some instances systemic antibiotics may be necessary. A clear diagnosis of invasive infection is important for the correct choice of antimicrobial to be used. Guidelines on the control of MRSA recommend that a sample of pus or tissue be taken from the site in order to gain a comprehensive diagnosis. Once treatment has commenced the patient is encouraged to have a daily bath or wash using a chlorhexidine-based soap for five days. Antiseptic hand and body washes are recommended for both the person caring for the patient and the infected patient, e.g. chlorhexidine, povidone-iodine, or triclosan antiseptic hand wash (Working Party, 1998).

Q6.8 How is MRSA prevented?

The primary objective of infection control is the prevention of spread of infection (Working Party, 1998) and the single most important practice to prevent the spread of MRSA is hand washing, for both patients and staff (see Q1.2, 1.3). The patient with MRSA should be encouraged to practise good hygiene. Soap and water is usually sufficient for most procedures, but an antiseptic detergent may be preferred.

In addition to good hand washing by staff, disposable gloves and aprons should be used when attending to dressings, performing aseptic techniques or dealing with blood and body fluids (Duckworth and Heathcock, 1995) (see Q1.4, 1.5, 1.14). Cuts or breaks in the skin of staff should be covered with an impermeable dressing in order to prevent the risk of infection. To ensure a high standard of infection control, continuing education of all staff in infection control is essential. When a patient with MRSA is discharged from, or transferred between, hospitals or from hospital to nursing home or vice versa it is good practice for staff to inform each other so that the necessary action can be taken. A patient attending an outpatient appointment should inform the staff that he or she is being treated for MRSA infection.

Q6.9 What is the risk to healthcare staff?

MRSA does not pose a risk to healthcare staff, family members of an affected patient or their close social or work contacts.

Q6.10 How should infected material such as dressings be disposed of in the community?

Clinical waste from a patient with MRSA should be disposed of in accordance with recommendations on the disposal of clinical waste (Health and Safety Commission, 1999) (see Q1.11, Q6.11).

Q6.11 What is clinical waste?

'Clinical waste consists wholly or partly of human or animal tissue, blood or other body fluids, excretions, swabs or dressings, syringes, needles or other sharp instruments, being waste which, unless rendered safe, may prove hazardous to any person coming into contact with it; and any other waste arising from medical, nursing, dental, veterinary, pharmaceutical or similar practice, investigation, treatment, care, teaching or research, or the collection of blood for transfusion, being waste which may cause infection to any person coming into contact with it' (Health and Safety Commission, 1999) (see Table 6.1).

Table 6.1 Clinical waste

Clinical waste is:
- Human tissue
- Any items that are or may be soiled by blood or other body fluids, for example
  - Wound dressings
  - Swabs
  - Disposable gloves and aprons
  - Materials used to clean up spillages (excluding cytotoxic spillages)
  - Colostomy and urine bags
  - Incontinence pads
  - Vomit bowls and sputum pots
  - Empty intravenous bags and administration sets
  - Sharps
  - Waste arising from treatment using cytotoxic drugs
  - Pharmaceutical waste – return all unused drugs to pharmacy

Clinical waste is not:
- Radioactive waste
- Flowers
- Newspapers
- Packaging
- Office waste
- Kitchen waste
- Apple cores
- Cans
- Bottles
- Aerosols

Source: Health and Safety Commission (1999).

The Health and Safety Commission recommends that all clinical waste is disposed of in an approved container, then transported for incineration or landfill in accordance with guidelines from the Health and Safety Commission and local policy.

Where healthcare staff treat patients in the home, employees have a duty to ensure that clinical waste generated is disposed of safely. Arrangements for disposal may be made through an employer's own system, or by special arrangement with the local collection authority.

Q6.12 Can dirty dressings be disposed of in the dustbin?

Dirty dressings that are clinical waste should be disposed of in yellow bags.

Q6.13 Are there special precautions to be taken within general practice?

Patients known to have MRSA-infected wounds should have the wound cared for at the end of surgery to reduce the risk of cross-infection. Universal precautions should be observed (see Q1.14). The clinical area should then be cleaned using disinfectant and water and dried thoroughly.

Q6.14 Should community healthcare staff have routine nasal/throat swabs following care of a patient with MRSA?

Community healthcare staff do not need routine nasal/throat swabs following care of a patient with MRSA (Working Party, 1998). Transient hand carriage in healthcare workers is well documented and staff should be encouraged to wash hands thoroughly between patients (see Q1.2, Figure 1.1). If there is a sudden increase in the number of community-acquired MRSA cases the Community Infection Control Nurse may investigate healthcare staff caring for the MRSA-infected patients.

Q6.15 Is it necessary to swab a wound after treatment?

If the patient is showing signs of infection in, for example, a leg ulcer or pressure sore then antibiotic therapy will normally be prescribed, as recommended by the microbiologist at the local hospital.

Currently the usual recommendation is to apply topical (mupirocin 2%) treatment for five days. This may not be appropriate if:

• the wound is large;
• the patient has had a recent course of mupirocin 2%;

- the MRSA is resistant to mupirocin 2%;
- the infection is in the urine.

In these situations advice should be sought from a microbiologist.

After five days of treatment and a further period of 48 hours the wound should be reassessed. If the wound has healed no further swabs, treatment or precautions are required. If the wound has not healed a further swab from the site of infection should be taken to ensure that the MRSA has cleared. If the swab is negative the precautions can be stopped. One negative swab is adequate in the community unless the patient needs to go into hospital, where the consultant may request three clear negatives.

Q6.16 What should I do if a patient has repeated MRSA infection?

If the site remains positive, MRSA precautions should be continued and the treatment recommenced on the advice of a microbiologist. Staff should observe wounds that have previously been infected with MRSA for signs of deterioration and if the site shows signs of infection a swab should be taken. Routine screening is not recommended.

Case history 12

An elderly female patient is discharged from hospital, having been admitted following a fall at home. She has had a small chronic leg ulcer for a number of years and is visited by the district nursing team twice a week for wound dressing. The wound does heal periodically but has recently started to deteriorate. The district nurse notes that the wound is now looking inflamed, red and is oozing discoloured fluid. The patient is complaining that the area feels hot to touch and has been painful over the past two or three days.

Action

The nurse suspects that there may be an infection and sends a wound swab to the local microbiology laboratory. The result shows infection with MRSA. The microbiologist recommends treatment with mupirocin 2% to be applied topically for five days. After the fifth day the wound begins to look a little better, it is no longer oozing, the inflammation is less apparent and the patient is no longer complaining of pain. On assessment of the wound the district nurse does not feel it necessary to re-swab the area as healing is taking place.

She stresses the importance of hand washing to the client. She continues to use an aseptic technique on the wound, and washes her hands in an antiseptic hand wash before and after caring for the wound. The patient lives alone, so there is no risk of cross-infection to other members of the household. However, the district nurse informs her colleagues that the patient has MRSA so that infection control, i.e. hand washing, remains a priority when caring for this patient.

For further information on wound infection and management, the reader is referred to Rainey, *Wound Management: A Handbook for Community Nurses*, in this series.

Impetigo

Q6.17 What is it?

Impetigo is a skin infection that most commonly causes small blisters which burst to form crusts on the face, arms or legs. Less commonly it causes much larger blisters known as 'bullae' on the face, buttocks, arms or legs.

Q6.18 What causes impetigo?

It is usually caused by *Staphylococcus aureus*, a bacterium that can colonize the nose (Darmstadt and Lane, 1994) (see Q6.2) or enter a break in the skin from a cut, puncture wound, vaccination site, insect bite, etc. (Cruickshank et al., 1982). However, *Streptococcus pyogenes* can also cause impetigo. It is possible to distinguish the organism only by microbiological identification (Brook et al., 1997).

Q6.19 How common is impetigo?

Impetigo is not a notifiable disease so there are no national figures available. It is more prevalent among children, in warm weather, crowded conditions (play groups, nurseries, etc.), where there is poor personal hygiene and where soap and water are not readily available (Chin, 2000) (see Q6.28).

Q6.20 What is the incubation period?

Probably four to 10 days (Chin, 2000).

Q6.21 How is it transmitted?

It is passed by direct contact with purulent skin lesions (Cruickshank et al., 1982), either spreading to other parts of the body (auto-infection) or being acquired by other people.

Q6.22 Who is at risk?

Anyone coming in direct contact with purulent skin lesions is at risk. Children tend to be at increased risk because of lack of hygiene, for example putting things in their mouth and not washing their hands. Spread within families is common because of close living conditions (see Q6.28). People with existing skin problems such as eczema or a scabies infection, where the integrity of the skin is already broken, are at most risk.

Q6.23 What are the signs and symptoms?

The initial lesions are pustules that produce a straw-coloured crust (Bielan, 1999). Eventually the crusts dry and fall off and the redness fades without scarring. The most common sites are the face, especially the nose and mouth, and limbs.

In bullous impetigo the initial lesion is less likely to rupture and the contents of the bullae can be observed to change from a clear to a cloudy fluid. When the bullae rupture, brown crusts are formed (Champion et al., 1998).

Q6.24 What is the natural history of the disease?

In some cases the infection will eventually clear up on its own (Robles, 1998). However, treatment will speed recovery and reduce the period of infection and therefore the potential for cross-infection (see Q6.27).

Q6.25 Can you get the infection twice?

Yes, previous infection does not provide immunity.

Q6.26 How is it diagnosed?

Diagnosis is by observation of the lesions and clinical history (e.g. other cases in the family, outbreak at school). Crusting of skin is very characteristic (see Q6.23). Identification of the causative organism is through culture of the lesion swab in the laboratory (Robles, 1998).

Q6.27 What is the treatment for impetigo?

Topical fusidic acid or mupirocin or, if infection is widespread, oral flucloxacillin or erythromycin is recommended (BNF, 2001). To aid topical treatment the crust should be gently washed off before application of the ointment.

Q6.28 How is it prevented?

The spread of impetigo is controlled through good personal hygiene and rapid identification and treatment of infected individuals. When advising a family about prevention of spread within the home it is important to highlight that they should observe good hygiene, not share towels and face flannels and avoid, where possible, direct contact with the lesions. Hands should be washed and dried thoroughly after applying topical treatment.

Infected children should be excluded from school until they have had 48 hours of antibiotic treatment or, if no antibiotics, the lesions are dried and healed. Outbreaks in residential settings such as nursing homes, schools and military establishments should be reported to the local public health department.

Q6.29 What are the implications for healthcare workers?

Staff should ensure that they wear protective gloves if dealing with lesions, and wash their hands well after removing their gloves (see Q1.4).

Staff who have impetigo infection should remain off work until the lesions are dry and healed, or they have had 48 hours of antibiotic treatment.

Case history 13

A school nurse is contacted by the head teacher of a local primary school. A number of children in the nursery at the school have been told they have impetigo by their GP. What advice should the head give to parents?

Action

If there are a number of children with symptoms of impetigo it would be a good idea to inform all parents what to do. (This is not recommended for isolated cases). The plan of action should be as follows:

1. *Inform parents about the increased numbers of children with impetigo.*
2. *Give parents information about impetigo, i.e. what it is, what causes it and how it can be contracted.*

3. *Exclude infected children until they have had 48 hours of antibiotic treatment.*
4. *Ensure paper towels and liquid soap are available for all staff and pupils (reusable towels and bar soap not recommended).*
5. *Inform the local public health department so that they can advise further.*

Shingles

Q6.30 What is shingles?

Shingles is caused by the same virus that causes chickenpox: the *Varicella zoster* virus. Chickenpox is a flu-like illness with fever and a characteristic rash, which is usually acquired during childhood. Most people recover between 10 and 15 days after the first few spots appear and usually get lifelong immunity. After an attack of chickenpox the virus lies dormant in the dorsal root ganglia (Chin, 2000).

Q6.31 What causes shingles?

The dormant virus, after a variable but usually long period, reactivates to cause shingles. Certain trigger factors such as stress, illness, shock or sometimes medical treatment are known to reactivate the virus.

Q6.32 How common is shingles?

Shingles is generally a disease of the elderly and over half the population will have had it by the age of 85 years (Griffiths, 2001). Although more common in the elderly it can occur in children, especially in immunosuppressed individuals.

Q6.33 What are the symptoms of shingles?

As the virus infects the nerve, it can cause severe pain. After two or three days the virus reaches the skin and causes painful blisters in a narrow band on one side of the body or face. For about a week new blisters will appear, which will be itchy and painful before drying out to form scabs. The whole episode normally takes between two and three weeks. However, some people will continue to have pain lasting six months or more (post-herpetic neuralgia). It is possible to have shingles anywhere on the body although the rash most commonly appears on the chest and abdominal areas. The commonest distribution of zoster rash is along the skin supplied by the intercostal nerve or over the face innervation of the ophthalmic branch of the trigeminal nerve. Severe ophthalmic zoster can permanently damage the cornea (Donaldson and Donaldson, 2000).

Q6.34 What are the complications of shingles?

Most patients will recover within a month. The commonest complication is post-herpetic neuralgia, which may last for six months or more in 30 per cent of the elderly (see Q6.33). Although most patients experience only one attack during their lifetime, multiple attacks may be seen in immunocompromised people.

Q6.35 Is shingles infectious?

The blisters of shingles may contain active virus. However, you cannot catch shingles from shingles nor can shingles be caught directly from someone with chickenpox. It is possible, though, for chickenpox to be caught from close contact with shingles blisters.

Q6.36 How can you prevent getting chickenpox from somebody with shingles?

To stop the spread of the virus avoid close contact with other people. As long as the blisters are covered the risk is minimal.

Q6.37 How is shingles diagnosed?

Diagnosis of shingles is usually made by a previous history of chickenpox and symptoms of a painful characteristic rash in a dermatome pattern (see Q6.33).

Q6.38 How is shingles treated?

The main thrust in managing shingles is providing supportive and symptomatic relief (see Box 6.1). A specific treatment for shingles is therapy with anti-viral agents. Acyclovir is licensed for treatment of shingles but is effective in reducing the incidence and severity of chronic pain only if given within the first 72 hours of onset of rash (Griffiths, 2001).

Box 6.1 Supportive and symptomatic treatment of shingles

1. Do not touch the rash as it could become infected and may take longer to heal
2. The blisters in shingles may contain active virus. To stop spread avoid close contact with other people
3. Wear loose-fitting clothes to ease the pressure of rubbing on the rash
4. Cooling the rash with ice cubes (wrapped in a flannel) or a cool bath may help
5. A soothing lotion like calamine may also bring relief
6. Rest and eat a good diet
7. Provide analgesics to combat pain

Q6.39 How can I avoid getting shingles?

You can avoid getting shingles only if you have not had chickenpox. There is a vaccine against chickenpox which has been licensed in the United Kingdom. Chickenpox is considered a mild disease from which most children recover, complications are few and the disease gives you lifelong immunity. Universal immunization of children against chickenpox is not being considered at present in the UK (DoH, 1996a) although some experts are recommending a routine screening and vaccination programme in pregnancy (Steadman et al., 1996).

Q6.40 Why is it necessary to protect pregnant women from chickenpox?

Chickenpox during pregnancy may result in stillbirth or congenital varicella syndrome, characterized by eye defects, limb hypoplasia, skin lesions and neurological abnormalities. The majority of the population get chickenpox during childhood, therefore the risk is limited. However, if a pregnant woman has not had chickenpox and is exposed then she will need investigating and protecting with immunoglobulin if found to be non-immune. The greatest risk is between 13 and 20 weeks of pregnancy (Enders et al., 1994), less so earlier and later.

Case history 14

A 28-year-old pregnant woman seeks advice from the GP because she has been looking after her 73-year-old grandmother who has been diagnosed with shingles. She wonders whether she has put her baby at risk.

Action

Infection with Varicella zoster *virus in pregnancy may result in a risk to the unborn child. The first thing to establish is whether she had chickenpox as a child. If that is the case then there is no risk. If she cannot remember whether she had chickenpox as a child, a blood test for antibodies to confirm previous infection can be done by the local microbiology laboratory. If the test shows that she has not had chickenpox in the past there is a need to find out what the risk is. The risk is present only if the blisters from her grandmother's shingles are wet and she has touched them. If the blisters have been covered and she has had no contact then the risk is extremely limited and nothing needs to be done. However, if the blood test confirms she has not had chickenpox in the past and she has touched infectious blisters the use of human* Varicella zoster *immunoglobulin (VZIG) should be considered. In terms of risk from a shingles patient, this should be used only when exposure occurs between 13 and 20 weeks as supplies of VZIG are limited. VZIG is prepared from blood-pooled plasma of blood donors with a history of recent chickenpox, which will protect the pregnant woman from developing chickenpox during pregnancy. VZIG is available from a local public health laboratory. In such situations, when pregnant women ask for advice in relation to risk to their baby from infections, expert guidance should be sought.*

Meningitis and Meningococcal Disease

Q6.41 What is meningitis?

Meningitis means inflammation of the lining of the brain, i.e. the meninges. Viruses are the most frequent cause of meningitis, followed by bacteria. Meningitis can also be caused by fungi, although this is uncommon and occurs mainly in immunocompromised patients. The signs of meningitis (or meningism) may also be produced by malignant cells, blood (following subarachnoid haemorrhage) or chemicals (drugs or contrast medium). Regardless of the agent causing meningitis, the signs and symptoms may be indistinguishable, especially early in the illness.

Viral meningitis

Viral meningitis (also known as aseptic meningitis) is a self-limiting condition that usually lasts between four and 10 days. Although in some cases there may be delay, recovery is usually complete.

Bacterial meningitis

Bacterial meningitis is a life-threatening disease and the most common causal agent is *Neisseria meningitides*, followed by *Streptococcus pneumoniae* (see

Q6.42). Until the early 1990s *Haemophilus influenza* type B (Hib) was an important cause of bacterial meningitis in young children. However, this disease has now been virtually eradicated from the United Kingdom by the introduction of Hib vaccine in 1992 (Cartwright et al., 1994).

Q6.42 What is the cause of meningococcal infection?

Neisseria meningitides is the cause of meningococcal infection, which can present as meningitis or septicaemia or a combination of the two. *Neisseria meningitides* is classified under a number of groups: the most common in England and Wales are group B (60 per cent) and group C (40 per cent) (see Box 6.2).

Box 6.2 Meningococcal Reference Unit: laboratory-confirmed Neisseria meningitides, England and Wales, by group, 1989–99 (mid-year totals)

	Group B	Group C	Other groups	Ungrouped	Total
1989–90	1019	477	37	2	1535
1990–91	964	422	39	6	1431
1991–92	938	329	39	3	1309
1992–93	878	320	42	6	1246
1993–94	822	311	46	6	1185
1994–95	871	307	51	11	1240
1995–96	872	618	65	0	1555
1996–97	1060	753	86	422	2321
1997–98	1099	775	112	308	2294
1998–99	1400	954	103	320	2777
1999/2000**	1627	889	148	133	2797

Note: **Provisional data.
Source: PHLS Meningococcal Reference Unit.

Q6.43 How common is meningococcal infection?

In recent years there has been an increase in the number of meningococcal infections in England and Wales (see Box 6.2). However, the introduction of immunization against meningococcal C disease in 1999 has led to a significant decrease in the number of cases. Meningococcal infection increases during winter (DoH, 1996a). The incidence of meningococcal infection is highest amongst children, especially infants and those under 5 years (Jones and Kaczmarski, 1995) followed by teenagers. Most cases are sporadic and occasionally there are two or more link cases (Stuart et al., 1997).

Q6.44 What is the incubation period?

The incubation period is between two and 10 days.

Q6.45 How is meningococcal infection transmitted?

Transmission is from the upper respiratory tract through prolonged and close contact (coughing, sneezing, intimate kissing).

Q6.46 Do some people carry meningococcal bacteria?

Meningococci can be found naturally at the back of the throat or nose. About 10 per cent of the general population carry one of a number of meningococcal strains, many of which are not virulent (Cartwright et al., 1987). Pathogenic strains of meningococci are found only in 1 per cent or so of carriers. These can be passed on to other individuals by droplet. Invasion of the blood and meninges by meningococci is not fully understood and it is not known why some individuals become ill while others stay well.

Q6.47 What are the symptoms of meningococcal infection?

The symptoms amongst infants and older children vary (see Box 6.3).

Q6.48 How quickly do symptoms develop?

With septicaemic illness, symptoms may develop over hours and the patient may be seriously ill. Symptoms of meningitis are variable and may take two or three days to develop.

Q6.49 How is meningococcal infection diagnosed?

The diagnosis of meningococcal infection is made by history of symptoms, examining clinical signs and confirmatory microbiological tests. Any general practitioner suspecting meningitis following clinical examination should administer benzylpenicillin IV or IM and refer the patient to a hospital immediately (see Q6.51). Within the hospital confirmatory tests will include changes in the blood and cerebrospinal fluid (presence of white cells, in particular an increase in polymorphs) and isolation of *Neisseria meningitides*. Further confirmation can be obtained by specialist laboratories using a polymerase chain reaction test.

Box 6.3 Clinical presentation of meningitis and/or septicaemia

Infants	Older children and adults
Non-specific	Non-specific
• Drowsiness	• Vomiting
• Irritability	• Fever
• Off feeds	• Back or joint pains
• Distress on handling	• Headache
• Vomiting or diarrhoea	
• Fever	
More specific	More specific
• Neck stiffness	• Neck stiffness
• Tense or bulging fontanelle	• Photophobia
• Purpuric or petechial rash that does not blanch under pressure	• Confusion
	• Purpuric or petechial rash that does not blanch under pressure
Late	Late
• High-pitched or moaning cry	• Coma
• Coma	• Shock
• Neck retraction	• Widespread haemorrhagic rash
• Shock	
• Widespread haemorrhagic rash	

Q6.50 If the meningitis is viral will the cerebrospinal fluid be clear?

The fluid may be clear or there may be increase in white blood cells, predominantly lymphocytes.

Q6.51 How is meningococcal infection treated?

Early antibiotic treatment is important in managing a case. GPs suspecting meningococcal infection should immediately give benzylpenicillin IM or IV (see Box 6.4) and transfer the patient to hospital. Giving penicillin early has been shown to improve prognosis (Cartwright et al., 1992;

Box 6.4 Benzylpenicillin dosage

Adult/child (10 years or over)	1200 mg IM or IV
Child (1–9 years)	600 mg IM or IV
Child (less than 1 year)	300 mg IM or IV

Strang and Pugh, 1992). Treatment in hospital will include nursing and medical support and specific therapy with a combination of antibiotics including penicillin and cephalosporins.

Q6.52 What is the natural history of meningococcal infection?

The overall mortality rate for meningococcal infection is around 10 per cent (PHLS, 1995c) rising to 50–60 per cent in children who present with meningococcal septicaemia and shock. One person in seven is left with a permanent disability, hearing loss being the most common.

Q6.53 When a case of meningococcal infection occurs is there a risk to others?

Close family contacts, i.e. those living in the same house, are at a slightly increased risk of infection as compared with the general population. Mouth-to-mouth contact, i.e. kissing, is also considered a close contact. These contacts should be given chemoprophylaxis to reduce the risk (PHLS, 1995c). Chemoprophylaxis is given to reduce carriage of meningococci among close family contacts and this should include the index case as well (see Box 6.5).

Box 6.5 Drug regime following menigococcal disease				
Age	*Antibiotic*	*Recommended dosage*	*Frequency*	*Route*
Chemoprophylaxis				
Baby <1 year	Rifampicin	5 mg/kg body weight	Every 12 hours for 2 days	Oral
Child	Rifampicin	10 mg/kg body weight	Every 12 hours for 2 days	Oral
Adult	Rifampicin	600mg	Every 12 hours for 2 days	Oral
Alternative chemoprophylaxis				
Child	Obtain further advice – Ciprofloxacin not licensed for children			
Adult	Ciprofloxacin	500 mg	Single dose (not licensed for this indication)	Oral

Q6.54 Are healthcare workers at increased risk?

There is no increased risk for healthcare workers who are involved in care of patients with meningococcal infection unless they have had mouth-to-mouth contact, i.e. resuscitation. If there has been mouth-to-mouth contact they will require chemoprophylaxis.

Q6.55 What if a meningococcal infection case arises in a nursery?

There is no need to provide chemoprophylaxis to all other children in the nursery. The risk of a secondary case in a nursery is no more than in the general population

Q6.56 What if there are two or more associated cases in the same school?

If such a situation arises the local consultant in communicable disease control or infection control nurse should be notified immediately. In such linked cases an outbreak control team will need to investigate and manage the situation (Barker et al., 1999).

Q6.57 What else can be done by community staff?

A case of meningococcal infection usually causes concern amongst residents of the local population. Continuing education of the public is important. Often the cases occur in a school. It is usual for local public health departments to contact the school to send a letter out to other parents informing them of the situation and reminding them of the need to identify symptoms early and seek medical help. Leaflets on meningitis are available from a variety of sources.

Summary

Community nurses need to be aware of the signs and symptoms of common respiratory diseases. The nurse may be the first point of contact for the patient, in either a clinic or home setting, and he or she requires the knowledge and resources to advise and support the patient and family. All staff have a responsibility to encourage influenza vaccination for vulnerable patients but need to offer unbiased information about the vaccine and side-effects, as with all vaccines. Although school nurses are usually involved in TB vaccination programmes, all staff may be asked questions about local policies. Nurses should be aware of their local programmes, where the local chest clinic is based, and the name of the contact nurse. The CCDC team is an invaluable resource during scares for meningitis or other infectious diseases.

Appendix 1

Disease	Usual incubation period	Period of communicability	Minimum period of exclusion of patients from school, day nursery, playgroup	Exclusion of family contacts who attend playgroup, day nursery or school
Gastrointestinal illness				
Campylobacter infection	1–11 days 2 days (usually 2–5)		Until clinically fit with no diarrhoea for at least 24 hours.	
Cryptosporidiosis	3–11 days (usually 2–5 days)	While organism is present in stools, but mainly until diarrhoea is present	Depending on the cause, children attending nursery/playgroup may be excluded for longer periods. Further advice from Consultants in Communicable Disease Control (CCDC).	Exclusion not necessary for any contact or family member of the index case. However, if symptoms develop, they should also be excluded until clinically fit with no diarrhoea for at least 24 hours
Dysentery	12 hours–7 days (usually 1–3 days)			
Salmonella food poisoning	12–72 hours			
Giardiasis	5–25 days (usually 7–10 days)	While cysts are present in stools, but mainly until diarrhoea is present	In rare cases, exclusion may be extended and negative stool specimens required. This will be at the discretion of the CCDC	
Hepatitis A (infective hepatitis)	2–6 weeks (usually 28–30 days)	From 7–14 days before to 7 days after onset of jaundice	7 days from onset of jaundice and when clinically fit with no symptoms	None
Paratyphoid fever	1–3 weeks	While organism is present in stools or urine	At the discretion of the CCDC	At the discretion of the CCDC
Typhoid fever	1–3 weeks	While organism is present in stools or urine	At the discretion of the CCDC	At the discretion of the CCDC
E-coli 0157 (VTEC)	1–6 days	While organism is present in stools	Seek advice from CCDC	Seek advice from CCDC

(contd)

Disease	Usual incubation period	Period of communicability	Minimum period of exclusion of patients from school, day nursery, playgroup	Exclusion of family contacts who attend playgroup, day nursery or school
Gastrointestinal illness				
Worms	Variable	Until worms have been treated	Until treated	Family members may require treatment
General infections				
Chickenpox	15–18 days	From 1–2 days before and up to 5 days after the appearance of rash	5 days from onset of rash (until spots are dry)	None
Conjunctivitis (viral or bacterial)	Depends on cause	While symptoms persist	Until treatment has begun and inflammation has started to resolve	None
Fifth disease (slapped cheek syndrome)	6–14 days	Not well known – mainly a few days before appearance of rash	Until clinically well	None
German measles (rubella)	14–21 days	About 7 days before to 4–5 days after onset of rash	5 days from appearance of rash	None
Glandular fever	28–42 days	Prolonged infectiousness, but once symptoms have subsided, risk is small apart from very close contact, e.g. kissing	Until clinical recovery	None
Hand, foot and mouth disease	3–5 days	Usually while symptoms persist	Until clinically well	None
Measles	10–15 days	A few days before to 4 days after onset of rash	5 days from onset of rash	None
Meningococcal disease (meningitis and septicaemia)	2–10 days (commonly 2–5 days)	While organism is present in nose and mouth	Until clinical recovery. CCDC will advise	No exclusion for contact receiving antibiotic prophylaxis

Disease	Usual incubation period	Period of communicability	Minimum period of exclusion of patients from school, day nursery, playgroup	Exclusion of family contacts who attend playgroup, day nursery or school
General infections				
Mumps	12–21 days	From a few days before onset of symptoms to subsidence of swelling (often 10 days)	Five days from onset of swollen glands	None
Scarlet fever and other streptococcal infections	1–3 days	While organism is present in the nasopharynx or skin lesion	Until clinical recovery or 48 hours after starting antibiotics	None
Tuberculosis	25–90 days	While organism is present in sputum. Usually non-infectious 2 weeks after starting treatment	CCDC will advise	Screening of contacts is routine policy in cases of pulmonary TB
Whooping cough (Pertussis)	10–14 days	7 days after exposure to 21 days after onset of paroxysmal coughing	21 days from onset of paroxysmal coughing or 5 days after commencing antibiotics	None

Skin infections
Good hand washing is essential if the spread of skin infection is to be reduced. Items such as towels and clothing must not be shared.

Disease	Usual incubation period	Period of communicability	Minimum period of exclusion of patients from school, day nursery, playgroup	Exclusion of family contacts who attend playgroup, day nursery or school
Impetigo (streptococcus pyogenes and staphylococcus aureus)	Usually 4–10 days, but can occur several months after colonization	While lesions remain moist or until 48 hours after starting antibiotic	Until 48 hours after starting antibiotic. Treatment is rapidly effective	None unless they show any signs of infection
Pediculosis capitis (head lice)	Lice eggs hatch in a week and reach maturity in 8–10 days	As long as eggs or lice remain alive	Until after treatment has been undertaken	Examination of family is required and treatment undertaken if necessary

(contd)

Disease	Usual incubation period	Period of communicability	Minimum period of exclusion of patients from school, day nursery, playgroup	Exclusion of family contacts who attend playgroup, day nursery or school
Skin infections				
Ringworm of the feet (athlete's foot)	Unknown	As long as lesions are present	Exclusion from school or barefoot exercise not necessary once treatment has commenced	None unless they show signs of infection
Ringworm of the scalp	10–14 days	As long as active lesions are present	Exclude until treatment has commenced	None unless they show signs of infection
Ringworm of the body	4–10 days	As long as lesions are present	Exclude until treatment has commenced	None unless they show signs of infection
Scabies	2–6 weeks, but with re-exposure only 1–4 days	Until eggs and mites are destroyed	Exclude until treatment has completed	Close contacts, i.e. family, will need treating at the same time as they may be incubating scabies.
Verrucae plantaris (plantar warts)	2–3 months, range 1–20 months	Unknown, probably as long as lesion visible	Not necessary. No evidence that wearing of verrucae socks during swimming prevents trans- mission to others	None

CCDC = Consultant in communicable disease control.

Resources

- For publications, support and research data on all aspects of liver disease:

British Liver Trust
Ransomes Europark
Ipswich 1PS 9QE, UK
Tel: 01473 276326; fax: 01473 276327; www.britishlivertrust.org.uk

- Special interest group for nurses (annual subscription £12):

British Liver Trust Nurses Forum
PO Box 900
Ipswich 1P3 9QW, UK.
Tel: 01473 276326.

- Information on occupational health and safety:

Health and Safety Executive (HSE)
Information Centre
Broad Lane
Sheffield S3 7HQ, UK.
Tel: 08701 545500 (info line); fax: 02920 859260; www.hse.gov.uk

- Special interest group for nurses:

HIV and AIDS Nursing National Forum
Royal College of Nursing
20 Cavendish Square
London W1M 0AB, UK
Tel: 0207 647 3740

- Detection, diagnosis and monitoring of communicable diseases. Contact for facts on diseases, publications and guidelines:

Public Health Laboratory Service (PHLS)
61 Colindale Avenue
London NW9 5DF, UK
Tel: 020 8200 1295; fax: 020 8200 8130/31; www.phls.co.uk

- Infection Control Nurses Association (ICNA)

Community Branch
Fitwise
Drumcross Hall
Bathgate
West Lothian
EH48 4BR
01506 811077
www.icna.co.uk

References

Ahmed AH, Nicholson KG, Nguyen-Van-Tam JS (1995) Reduction in mortality associated with influenza vaccine during 1989–90 epidemic. *Lancet* 346: 591–5.

Allwright S, Bradley F, Long J, Barry J, Thornton L, Parry JV (1999) Prevalence of antibodies to Hepatitis B, Hepatitis C, and HIV and risks factors in Irish prisoners: results of a national cross sectional survey. *British Medical Journal* 321: 78–82.

Ashley J, Smith T, Dunnell K (1996) Deaths in Great Britain associated with the influenza epidemic of 1989/90. *Population Trends OPCS* London: Stationery Office 5: 16–20.

Aston R, Duggal H, Simpson J (1998) Head Lice: Report for Consultants in Communicable Disease Control (C'sCDC). The Public Health Medicine Environmental Group Executive Committee [Available at: www.http://fam-english.demon.co.uk/phmeghl.htm].

Ayliffe GAJ, Lowbury EJL, Geddes AM and Williams JD (eds) (1992) *Control of Hospital Infection: A Practical Handbook*. London: Chapman & Hall Medical.

Barker RM, Shakespeare RM, Mortimore AJ, Allen NA, Solomon CL, Stuart JM (1999) Practical guidelines for responding to an outbreak of meningococcal disease among university students based on experience in Southampton. *Communicable Disease and Public Health* 2(3): 168–73.

Barrett NJ, Morse DL (1993) The Resurgence of Scabies. Communicable Disease Report. *CDR Review*: R32–34.

Barwell R, Shields S (1997) Deaths associated with Ivermectin treatment of scabies. *Lancet* 349: 1144–5.

Bielan B (1999) What's your assessment? *Dermatology Nursing* 11(5): 354–5.

Bouchier I (1998) *Cryptosporidium in Water Supplies. Report of the Group of Experts: Department of the Environment, Transport and the Regions and Department of Health*. London: HMSO.

Bowell B (1992) A risk to others. *Nursing Times* 88(4): 38–40.

Boyce TG, Swerdlow DL, Griffin PM (1995) Escherichia Coli 0157: H7 and the haemolytic–uraemic syndrome. *New England Journal of Medicine* 10 August: 364–8.

Brettle R (2001) Natural history of HIV/AIDS. *Medicine: HIV and AIDS* 29: 9–11.

British National Formulary (2000) London: British Medical Association and the Royal Pharmaceutical Society of Great Britain.

British National Formulary (2001) London: BMJ Books.

British Standards Institution (1990) *Specification for Sharps Containers*, BS 7320. London: British Standards Institution.

Brook I, Frazier EH, Yeager JK (1997) Microbiology of nonbullous impetigo. *Paediatric Dermatology* 14(3): 192–5.

Brown JS, Wells F, Duckworth G, Paul EA, Barnes NC (1995) Improving notification rates for tuberculosis. *British Medical Journal* 310: 974.

Burgess I (1996) Management guidelines for lice and scabies. *Prescriber* 7: 87–99.

Burgess IF (1990) Carbaryl lotions for head lice: new laboratory tests show variation in efficacy. *Pharmaceutical Journal* 245: 159–61.

Burgess IF (1995a) Head lice and their management. *Advances in Parasitology* 36: 271–343.

Burgess IF (1995b) Authors differ on assessment of flaws in trials. *British Medical Journal* 311: 1369.

Burgess IF, Veal L, Sindle T (1992) The efficacy of d-phenothrin and permethrin formulations against head lice: a comparison. *Pharmaceutical Journal* 249: 692–3.

Cafferkey MT, Hone R, Keane CT (1988) Sources and outcome for methicillin resistant staphylococcus aureus bacteraemia. *Journal of Hospital Infection* 11: 136–43.

Cartwright K, Reilly S, White D, Stuart J (1992) Early treatment with parenteral penicillin in meningococcal disease. *British Medical Journal* 305: 143–7.

Cartwright KAV, Begg NT, Rudd P (1994) Use of vaccines and antibiotic prophylaxis in contacts and cases of Haemophylus influenzae type B (Hib) disease. *Communicable Disease Report* 2: R16–R17.

Cartwright KAV, Stewart JM, Jones DM, Noah ND (1987) The Stonehouse Survey: nasopharyngeal carriage of meningococci and *Neisseria lactamica*. *Epidemiology of Infections* 99: 591–601.

CDSC (2000) AIDS and HIV infection in the United Kingdom: monthly report. *Communicable Disease Report Weekly* 10: 425–6.

Champion RH, Burton JL, Burns DA, Breathnach SM (1998) *Textbook of Dermatology*. London: Blackwell Science.

Chin J (2000) *Control of Communicable Diseases Manual* 17th edn. Washington, DC: American Public Health Association.

Chosidow O (2000) Scabies and pediculosis. *Lancet* 355: 819–26.

Chosidow O, Chastang C, Brue C, Bouvet E, Izri M, Monteny N, Bastuji-Gann S, Rousset J-J, Revuz J (1994) Controlled study of malathion and d-phenothrin lotions for pediculus humanus capitis: infested school children. *Lancet* 344: 1724–7.

Communicable Disease Report (2000a) Trends in selected gastrointestinal infection 1999. *Communicable Disease Report Weekly* 10 (January): 2, 9.

Communicable Disease Report (2000b) Outbreak of salmonellosis associated with chicks and ducklings at a children's nursery. *Communicable Disease Report Weekly* 10(April): 17, 149, 152.

Communicable Disease Surveillance Centre (1999) *Gastrointestinal Section. Annual Corrected Notifications, England and Wales 1949–1988 and 1989–1998*. London: CDSC.

Coyne PE, Addiss DG (1997) Deaths associated with Ivermectin for scabies. *Lancet* 350: 215–16.

Crowley DS, Ryan MJ, Wall PG (1997) Gastroenteritis in children under 5 years of age in England and Wales. *Communicable Disease Report Review* 7(6): R82–R86.

Cruickshank JG, Lightfoot NF, Sugars KH, Coleman G, Simmons MD, Tolliday J, Oakley EHN (1982) A large outbreak of streptococcal pyoderma in a military training establishment. *Journal of Hygiene* 89: 9–21.

Darmstadt GL, Lane AT (1994) Impetigo: an overview. *Paediatric Dermatology* 11(4): 293–303.

Del Guidice P, Marty P (1999) Ivermectin in elderly patients. *Archives of Dermatology* 135: 351–2.

Department of Health (1993) *Protecting Health Care Workers and Patients from Hepatitis B*, HSG (93)40. London: DoH.

Department of Health (1994) *HTM 2010: Transportable Sterilizers*, NHS Estates, Agency of the Department of Health. London: DoH.

Department of Health (1996a) *Immunisation against Infectious Disease*. London: HMSO.

Department of Health, Expert Working Party (1996b) *Food Handlers: Fitness to Work. Guidelines for Food Business Managers*. London: HMSO.

Department of Health (1997) *UK Health Departments' Contingency Plan for Pandemic Influenza. The Influenza Pandemic Plan*. London: DoH.

Department of Health (1998a) *Guidance for Clinical Health Care Workers: Protection against Infection with HIV and Hepatitis Viruses. Recommendations of the Expert Advisory Group on AIDS*. London: HMSO.

Department of Health (1998b) *Screening of Pregnant Women for Hepatitis B and Immunisation of Babies at Birth*, HSC 1998/127. London: DoH.

Department of Health (1998c) *AIDS/HIV Infected Health Care Workers: Guidance on the Management of Infected Health Care Workers and Patient Notification*. HSC 1998/226.

Department of Health (1999a) *Reducing Mother to Baby Transmission of HIV*, HSC 199/183. London: DoH.

Department of Health (1999b) *HIV and Infant Feeding Guidance from the UK Chief Medical Officer's Expert Advisory Group on AIDS*. London: DoH.

Department of Health (1999c) *Health Advice for Travellers*. London: HMSO.

Department of Health (2000) Major changes to the policy on influenza immunization. *CMO's Update 2000* 26: 1.

Djuretic T, Wall PG, Ryan MJ, Evans HS, Adak GK, Cowden JM (1996) General outbreaks of infectious intestinal disease in England and Wales 1992–1994. *Communicable Disease Report Review* 6(4): R57–R63.

Donaldson RJ, Donaldson LJ (2000) *Essential Public Health*. London: Kluwer.

Dore GJ, Kaldon JM, McCaughan W (1997) Systematic review of polymerase chain reaction in defining infectiveness amongst people infected with Hepatitis C virus. *British Medical Journal* 315: 333–7.

Downs AM, Harvey I, Kennedy CT (1999) The epidemiology of headlice and scabies in the UK. *Epidemiology and Infection* 122(3): 471–7.

Duckworth G, Heathcock R (1995) Report of a combined working party of the British Society for Antimicrobial Chemotherapy and the Hospital Infection Society. Guidelines on Control of methicillin resistant staphylococcus in the community. *Journal of Hospital Infection* 31: 1–12.

Duckworth GJ (1993) Diagnosis and management of methicillin resistant *Staphlococcus aureus* infection. *British Medical Journal* 307: 1049–52.

Duckworth GJ, Heptonstall J, Aitkin C for the Incident Control Team and others (1999) Transmission of Hepatitis C virus from a surgeon to a patient. *Communicable Diseases and Public Health* 2: 188–92.

EASL (1999) International Consensus Statement on Hepatitis C. *Journal of Hepatology* 30: 956–61.

Effectiveness Matters (1999) Treating headlice and scabies. *Effectiveness Matters* [University of York] 4(1).

Ejidokum OO, Killalea D, Cooper M, Holmyard S, Cross A, Kemp C (2000) Four linked outbreaks of *Salmonella enteritidis* phage type 4 infection: the continuing egg threat. *Communicable Disease and Public Health* 3(2): 95–100.

Enders G, Miller E, Crackock-Watson J, Bolley I, Ridehaigh M (1994) Consequences of Varicella and Herpes zoster in pregnancy: prospective study of 1739 cases. *Lancet* 343: 1548–50.

Environmental Protection Act (1990) *1996 Waste Management: The Duty of Care Code of Practice*. London: HMSO.

Evans HS, Madden P, Douglas C, Adak GK, O'Brien SJ, Djuretic T, Wall PG, Stanwell-Smith R (1998) General outbreaks of infectious intestinal disease in England and Wales 1995 and 1996. *Communicable Disease and Public Health* 1(3): 165–71.

Evans HS, Maguire H (1996) Outbreaks of infectious intestinal disease in schools and nurseries in England and Wales 1992–1994. *Communicable Disease Report Review* 6(7): R103–R108.

Figueroa J (1998) Scabies. In: *Primary Health Care Guide to Common UK Parasitic Diseases*. London: Community Hygiene Concern.

Fleming D, Charlton J, McCormick A (1997) The population at risk in relation to influenza immunization policy England and Wales. *Health Trends* 29(2): 42–7.

Fleming DM, Watson JM, Nicholas S, Smith GE, Swan AV (1995) Study of the effectiveness of influenza vaccination in the elderly in the epidemic of 1989–90 using a general practice database. *Epidemiology and Infection* 115: 581–9.

Foster GR, Goldin RD, Main J, Murray-Lyon I, Hargreaves S, Thomas HC (1997) Management of chronic Hepatitis C: clinical audit of biopsy based management algorithm. *British Medical Journal* 315: 453–8.

French GL, Cheng AFB, Ling, JML, Mo P, Donnan S (1990) Hong Kong strains of methicillin resistant and methicillin sensitive *Staphlococcus aureus* have similar virulence. *Journal of Hospital Infection* 15: 117–25.

Furtado C, Adak GK, Stuart JM, Wall PG, Evans HS, Casemore DP (1998) Outbreaks of waterborne infectious intestinal disease in England and Wales 1992–95. *Epidemiology and Infection* 121: 109–19.

Gay NJ, Morgan-Capner P, Wright J, Farrington CP, Miller E (1994) Age-specific antibody prevalence to hepatitis in England: implications for disease control. *Epidemiology and Infection* 112: 113–20.

Gazzard B, Moyle G, on behalf of the BHIVA Guidelines Writing Committee (1998) Revision to the British HIV Association guidelines for antiretroviral treatment of HIV seropositive individuals. *Lancet* 352: 314–16.

Griffiths PD (2001) Herpes viruses. *Medicine: Infections* 29: 112.

Guy's Hospital (1994) *Nursing Drug Reference* London: Mosby.

Hardie RM, Watson JM (1992) Mycobacterium bovis in England and Wales: past, present and future. *Epidemiology and Infection* 109: 23–31.

Hayward AC, Watson JM (1995) Tuberculosis in England and Wales 1982–1993: notifications exceed predictions. *Communicable Disease Report* 5(3): R29–R33.

Health and Safety Commission (1999) *Safe Disposal of Clinical Waste. Health and Safety Advisory Committee*. Norwich: HSE Books.

Health and Safety Executive (1992) *Personal Protective Equipment at Work: Guidance on Regulations*. London: HMSO.

Health and Safety Executive (1994) *Control of Substances Hazardous to Health Regulations*, revised. London: HMSO.

Health Service Advisory Committee (1999) *Safe Disposal of Clinical Waste*, 2nd edn. Norwich: Health and Safety Executive.

Health Service Circular (1999) Variant Creutzfeldt-Jakob Disease (VCJD): minimising the risk of transmission. HSC 1999/178 DoH.

Health Service Circular (1999) Controls Assurance in Infection Control: Decontamination of Medical Devices. HSC 1999/179 DoH.

Health Service Circular (2000) Decontamination of medical devices. HSC 2000/032. DoH.

Heptonstall J (1992) Outbreaks of hepatitis B virus infections associated with infected surgical staff. *Communicable Disease Report CDR Review* 1: R81–R85.

Hospital Infection Control (1996) Lab outbreak of *Shigella* spreads via faucet handles. *Hospital Infection Control* 23(11): 142–3.

HSG (1993) *Public Health: Responsibilities of the NHS and the Roles of Others.* HSG (93) 56.

HSG (1996) *Minor Surgery in General Practice: Guidance from the Medical Services Committee & the Royal College of General Practitioners.* HSG (93) 40.

Hudson S, Lightfoot N, Coulson J, Russell K, Sisson P, Sobo A (1991) Jackdaws and magpies as vectors of milkborne human Campylobacter infection. *Epidemiology and Infection* 107: 363–72.

Joint Committee of the British Thoracic Society (2000) Control and prevention of TB in the United Kingdom: Code of Practice 2000. *Thorax* 55: 887–901.

Jones DM, Kaczmarski EB (1995) Meningococcal infections in England and Wales: 1994. *Communicable Disease Report Review* 5: R125–R130.

Kendall EJC, Tanner EI (1982) Campylobacter enteritis in general practice. *Journal of Hygiene* 88: 155–63.

Lindsay S (1993) 200 years of lice in Glasgow: an index of social deprivation. *Parasitology Today* 9: 412–17.

Maguire H, Heptonstall J, Begg N (1992) The epidemiology and control of Hepatitis A. *Communicable Disease Report Review* 10: R114–R117.

Maguire H, Handford S, Perry K, Nicholas S, Waight P, Parry J, O'Mahony M, Begg N (1995) A collaborative case control study of sporadic hepatitis A in England. *Communicable Disease Report Review* 5(3): R33–R40.

Maguire HC, Seng C, Chambers S, Cheasty T, Double G, Soltanpoor N, Morse D (1998) Shigella outbreak in a school associated with eating canteen food and person to person spread. *Communicable Disease and Public Health* 1(4): 279–80.

Mandell G, Douglas R, Bennett J (1990) *Principles and Practice of Infectious Diseases*, 3rd edn. London: Churchill Livingstone.

Mangtani P, Heptonstill J, Hall AJ (1998) Enhanced surveillance of acute symptomatic hepatitis B in England and Wales. *Communicable Disease and Public Health* 1: 114–20.

McDonnell RJ, Wall PG, Adak GK, Evans HS, Cowden JM, Caul EO (1995) Outbreaks of infectious intestinal disease associated with person to person spread in hotels and restaurants. *Communicable Disease Report Review* 5(10): R150–R152.

McHutchison JG, Gordon SC, Schiff ER, Mitchell SL, Lee WM, Rustgi KR, Goodman ZD, Ling M, Cort S, Albrecht JK, for the Hepatitis Interventional Therapy Group (1998) Interferon alpha: 2b alone or in combination with ribavarin as initial treatment for chronic Hepatitis C. *New England Journal of Medicine* 339: 1485–92.

Mead PS, Griffin MP (1998) Escherichia coli O157: H7. *Lancet* 352: 1207–12.

Meers P, Sedgwick J, Worsley M (1995) *The Microbiology and Epidemiology of Infection for Health Science Students.* London: Chapman & Hall.

Meers PD, Ayliffe GAJ, Emmerson AM, Leigh DA, Mayon-White RT, Mackintosh CA, Stronge JL (1981) Report on the National survey of Infection in Hospitals, 1980. *Journal of Hospital Infection* 2(Suppl.).

Meheus A (1999) Report on the VHPB meeting in Nice, France, 25–27 March 1999: Israel implements universal hepatitis A immunization. *Viral Hepatitis* 8(1): 2.

Mims CA, Dimmock NJ, Nash A, Stephen J (1995) *Mims Pathogenesis of Infectious Disease*, 4th edn. London: Academic Press.

Mohle-Boetani JC, Stapleton M, Finger R, Bean N, Pundstone J, Blake PA, Griffin P (1995) Communitywide Shigellosis: control of an outbreak and risk factors in child day-care centers. *American Journal of Public Health* 85(6): 812–16.

Muncuoglu KY, Miller J, Gofin R, Alder B, Ben-Ishai F, Almog R, Klaus S (1990) Epidemiological studies on head lice infestation in Israel. *International Journal of Dermatology* 29: 502–6.

National Prescribing Centre (1999) The management of scabies and threadworms. *Prescribing Nurse Bulletin* 1: 3.

Newman CPS (1993) Surveillance and control of *Shigella sonnei* infection. *Communicable Disease Report Review* 3(5): R63–R68.

Nguyen-Van-Tam JS, Nicholson KG (1993) Influenza immunization: vaccine offer, request and uptake in high risk patients during the 1991/2 season. *Epidemiology and Infection* 111: 347–55.

NHS Centre for Reviews and Dissemination (1996) Influenza vaccination and older people. *Effectiveness Matters* 2(1).

Offidani A, Cellini A, Simonetti O, Fumelli C (1999) Treatment of scabies with Invermectin. *European Journal of Dermatology* 9(2): 100–1.

Old DC, Mather H, Cheasty T (2000) Family outbreak of dysentery caused by a rhamnose non-fermenting, ONPG-negative strain of *Shigella sonnei* phage type 6. *Communicable Disease and Public Health* 3(2): 135–6.

Parry J, Duggal H, Beaumont M, Jenkinson H, Price C (2001) A report of an outbreak of shigellosis in a primary school in Staffordshire. Public Health.

Parry J, Perry K, Mortimer P (1987) Sensitive assays of viral antibodies in saliva: an alternate to tests on serum. *Lancet* ii: 72–5.

Parry J, Perry K, Mortimer P, Farrington C, Waight P, Miller E (1988) Rational programme for screening travellers for antibodies to Hepatitis A virus. *Lancet* i: 1447–9.

Pebody RG, Ryan MJ, Wall PG (1997) Outbreaks of campylobacter infection: rare events for a common pathogen. *Communicable Disease Report Review* 7(3): R33–R37.

Pennington Report (1997) *The Pennington Group Report on the Circumstances leading to the 1996 outbreak of infection with* E. coli 0157 in Central Scotland: The Implications for Food and Safety and the Lessons to be Learned. Edinburgh: Stationery Office.

PHLS (1995a) Working Party of the PHLS Salmonella Committee. The prevention of human transmission of gastrointestinal infections, infestations, and bacterial intoxications: a guide for public health physicians and environmental health officers in England and Wales. *Communicable Disease Report Review* 5(11): R166.

PHLS (1995b) Sub-committee of the PHLS Working Group on vero cytotoxin producing *Escherichia coli* (VTEC): interim guidelines for the control of infections with vero cytotoxin producing *Escherichia coli* (VTEC). *Communicable Disease Report* 5(6): R77–R83.

PHLS (1995c) Meningococcal Infections Working Group & Public Health Medicine Environmental Group. Control of meningococcal disease: guidance for Consultants in Communicable Disease Control. *Communicable Disease Report Review* 5: R189–R195.

PHLS (2000a) Subcommittee of the PHLS Advisory Committee on Gastrointestinal Infections. Guidelines for the control of infection with vero cytotoxin producing *Escherichia coli* (VTEC). *Communicable Disease and Public Health* 3(1): 14–23.

PHLS (2000b) Lice and Scabies: A Health Professional's Guide to Epidemiology and Treatment. Colindale, London: Public Health Laboratory Service.

PHLS Hepatitis Subcommittee (1992) Exposure to Hepatitis B virus: guidance on post exposure prophylaxis. *Communicable Disease Report CDR Review* 2: R97–R101.

PHLS Working Group on the control of *Shigella sonnei* infection (1993) Revised guidelines for the control of *Shigella sonnei* infection and other infective diarrhoeas. *Communicable Disease Report* 3(5): R69–R70.

Piot P, Bartos M, Ghys PD, Walker N, Schwartlander B (2001) The global impact of HIV/AIDS. *Nature* 410: 968–73.

PoynardT, Marcellin P, Lee SS, Niederau C, Minuk GS, Ideal G, Bain V, Heathcote J, Zeuzem S, Threpo C, Albrecht JK for the International Hepatitis Interventional Therapy Group (1998) Randomised trial of interferon alpha 2b plus ribavirin for 48 weeks or for 24 weeks versus interferon alpha 2b plus placebo for 48 weeks for treatment of chronic infection with Hepatitis C virus. *Lancet* 352: 1426–32.

Ramsay ME, MA Balogun, Colins M, Balraj U (1998) Laboratory surveillance of Hepatitis C virus infection in England and Wales: 1992 to 1996. *Communicable Diseases and Public Health* 2: 89–94.

Reintjes R, Bosman A, de Zwart O, Stevens M, van der Knaap L, van den Hoek K (1999) Outbreak of hepatitis A in Rotterdam associated with visits to 'darkrooms' in gay bars. *Communicable Disease and Public Health* 2(1): 43–6.

Robles WS (1998) *Skin infections. In:* Managing Infections. Oxford: Bios Scientific Publishers.

Salisbury DM, Begg NT (1996) *Immunisation Against Infectious Disease.* London: HMSO.

Sanderson, PJ (1994) Common bacterial pathogens and resistance to antibiotics. *British Medical Journal* 289: 638–9.

Sin J, Quigley C, Davies M (2000) Survey of raw egg use by home caterers. *Communicable Disease and Public Health* 3(2): 90–4.

Sinclair A (1997) Tackling a visitation of threadworms. *Professional Care of Mother and Child* 7: 53–4.

Siu A (1994) Methicillin Resistant *Staphylococcus Aureus*: do we just have to live with it? *British Journal of Nursing* 3: 753–9.

Skirrow MB (1977) Campylobacter enteritis: a 'new' disease. *British Medical Journal* 2: 9-11.

Steadman DS, Stevenson DK, Arvin AM (1996) Variella vaccine in pregnancy: routine screening and vaccination should be considered. *British Medical Journal* 313: 701–2.

Stevenson J, Hanson S (1996) Outbreak of *Escherichia coli* 0157 phage type 2 infection associated with eating precooked meats. *Communicable Disease Report* 6(8): R116–R118.

Strang JR, Pugh EJ (1992) Meningococcal infections: reducing the case fatality rate by giving penicillin before admission to hospital. *British Medical Journal* 305: 141–3.

Stuart JM, Monk PN, Lewis DA, Constantine C, Kaczmarski EB, Cartwright KAV, on behalf of the PHLS Meningococcus Working Group and Public Health Medicine Environmental Group (1997) Management of clusters of meningococcal disease. *Communicable Disease Report* 7: R3–R5.

Stuart J, Majeed F, Cartwright K, Room R, Parry J, Perry K, Begg N (1992) Salivary antibody testing in a school outbreak of Hepatitis A. *Epidemiology and Infection* 109: 161–6.

Sundkvist T, Hamilton G, Houriham B, Hart I (2000) Outbreak of Hepatitis A spread by contaminated drinking glasses in a public house. *Communicable Disease and Public Health* 3(1): 60–2.

Taylor L (1990) Infection control at your fingertips: procedures for preventing and controlling MRSA. *Professional Nurse* 5(10): 547–71.

Teo CG (1992) The virology and serology of hepatitis: an overview. *Communicable Disease Report CDR Review* 2: R110–R114.

Tong MJ, El-Farra NS, Reikes AR, Co RL (1995) Clinical outcomes after transfusion associated Hepatitis C. *New England Journal of Medicine* 332: 1463–6.

Tweed P, Molineux C, Edwards M (1999) Ethics. In: Edwards M, ed. *The Informed Practice Nurse.* London: Whurr Publishers.

Van Damme P (1997 Integration of Hepatitis B vaccination into national immunisation programme. *British Medical Journal* 314: 1033–6.

Vander Stichele RH, Dezeure EM, Bogaert MG (1995) Systematic review of clinical efficacy of topical treatments for head lice. *British Medical Journal* 311: 604–812.

Vermaak Z (1996) Model for the control of pediculus humanus capitis. *Public Health* 110: 283–8.

Wall PG, de Louvois J, Gilbert RJ, Rowe B (1997) Food poisoning: notifications, laboratory reports and outbreaks: where do the statistics come from and what do they mean? *Communicable Disease Report Review* 6(7): R93–R100.

Wall PG, McDonnell RJ, Adak GK, Cheasty T, Smith HR, Rowe B (1996) General outbreaks of vero cytotoxin producing *Escherichia coli* O157 in England and Wales from 1992 to 1994. *Communicable Disease Report* 6(2): R26–R33.

Ward L (2000) Salmonella perils of pet reptiles. *Communicable Disease and Public Health* 3(1): 2–3.

Waugh N (1998) *Ribavarin and Interferon Alpha in the Treatment of Chronic Hepatitis C.* Aberdeen: Scottish Health Purchasing Information Centre

Wilson J (1995) *Infection Control in Clinical Practice.* London: Baillière-Tindall.

Winter GF (1999) *Clinical Virology: A Guide for Practitioners.* London: Nursing Times Books.

Working Party of the PHLS *Salmonella* Committee (1995) The prevention of human transmission of gastrointestinal infections, infestations and bacterial intoxications: a guide for public health physicians and environmental health officers in England and Wales. *Communicable Disease Report Review* 5(11): R167.

Working Party Report (1998) Revised guidelines for the control of methicillin-resistant *Staphylococcus aureus* infection in hospitals. *Journal of Hospital Infection* 39: 253–90.

Zuckerman M, Pillay D (2001) HIV Testing and Monitoring. *Medicine: HIV and AIDS* 29: 9–11.

Index